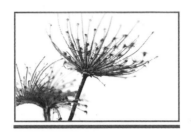

Culture, Heritage, and Diversity
in Older Adult Mental Health Care

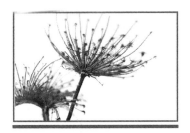

Culture, Heritage, and Diversity
in Older Adult Mental Health Care

Edited by

Maria D. Llorente, M.D., FAPA

APA Council on Geriatric Psychiatry

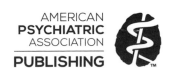

AMERICAN
PSYCHIATRIC
ASSOCIATION
PUBLISHING

If you wish to buy 50 or more copies of the same title, please go to www.appi.org/specialdiscounts for more information.

Copyright © 2019 American Psychiatric Association Publishing

ALL RIGHTS RESERVED

First Edition

Manufactured in the United States of America on acid-free paper
22 21 20 19 18   5 4 3 2 1

American Psychiatric Association Publishing
800 Maine Avenue, S.W.
Suite 900
Washington, DC 20024-2812
www.appi.org

Library of Congress Cataloging-in-Publication Data
Names: Llorente, Maria D., editor. | American Psychiatric Association
   Publishing, issuing body.
Title: Culture, heritage, and diversity in older adult mental health care/
   edited by Maria D. Llorente.
Description: First edition. | Washington, DC : American Psychiatric
   Association Publishing, [2019] | Includes bibliographical references.
Identifiers: LCCN 2018023367 (print) | LCCN 2018024976 (ebook) |
   ISBN 9781615372119 (ebook) | ISBN 9781615372058 (pbk. : alk. paper)
Subjects: | MESH: Health Services for the Aged—organization & administra-
   tion | Mental Health Services—organization & administration | Culturally
   Competent Care | Aged—psychology | Cultural Diversity | United States
Classification: LCC RC451.4.A5 (ebook) | LCC RC451.4.A5 (print) |
   NLM WT 31 | DDC 362.2084/6—dc23
LC record available at https://lccn.loc.gov/2018023367

British Library Cataloguing in Publication Data
A CIP record is available from the British Library.

Contents

1 Why Is Cultural Competency Important When Working With Older Adults?

Amy Gajaria, M.D., FRCPC
Ebony Dix, M.D.
Ken Sakauye, M.D.
Maria D. Llorente, M.D., FAPA

2 Cultural Competence in Geriatric Psychiatry Teaching and Evaluative Methods

Ken Sakauye, M.D.
Shuo Sally He, M.D., M.P.H.
Ebony Dix, M.D.
Raissa Tanqueco, M.D.
Iqbal Ahmed, M.D., FRCPsych

3 Migration, Acculturation, and Mental Health

Carl I. Cohen, M.D.
Pachida Lo, M.D.
Carine Nzodom, M.D.
Samra Sahlu, M.D.

Contributors

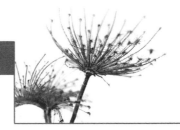

Iqbal Ahmed, M.D., FRCPsych
Faculty Psychiatrist, Tripler Army Medical Center; Professor of Psychiatry, Uniformed Services University of Health Sciences; Professor of Psychiatry and Geriatric Medicine, University of Hawai'i at Mānoa, Honolulu, Hawaii

Yasmin Banaei, M.D.
Psychiatry Resident, Medstar Georgetown University, Washington, D.C.

R. Dakota Carter, M.D.
Child and Adolescent Fellow, University of Texas Health Science Center, Houston, Texas

Carl I. Cohen, M.D.
SUNY Distinguished Professor and Director, Division of Geriatric Psychiatry, Department of Psychiatry, SUNY Downstate Medical Center, Brooklyn, New York

Ebony Dix, M.D.
PGY-4, Chief Resident, Department of Behavioral Medicine and Psychiatry, West Virginia University School of Medicine, Morgantown, West Virginia

Amy Gajaria, M.D., FRCPC
PGY-6 Resident, Child and Adolescent Psychiatry, University of Toronto, Toronto, Ontario, Canada

Jai C. Gandhi, M.D.
PGY-5 Resident and Consultation-Liaison Fellow, Department of Psychiatry, University of Washington, Seattle, Washington

Rita Hargrave, M.D.
Geriatric Psychiatrist, Northern California Health Care System, Martinez, California

Shuo Sally He, M.D., M.P.H.
Resident, Department of Psychiatry, George Washington University Hospital, Washington, D.C.

Vicenzio Holder-Perkins, M.D., M.P.H.
Chief of Psychiatry, Washington D.C. Veterans Affairs Medical Center; Assistant Clinical Professor, Department of Psychiatry and Behavioral Sciences, George Washington University, Washington, D.C.

Marilyn Horvath, M.D.
Staff Psychiatrist, Martinsburg West Virginia VA Medical Center, Martinsburg, West Virginia

Raya Elfadel Kheirbek, M.D., M.P.H.
Geriatrician and Palliative Care Physician, Washington DC VA Medical Center; Associate Professor of Medicine, School of Medicine and Health Sciences, George Washington University, Washington, D.C.

Shiv Lamba
Flint High School, Flint, Michigan

Maria D. Llorente, M.D., FAPA
Deputy Chief of Staff, Washington DC VA Medical Center, Department of Veterans Affairs; Professor of Psychiatry, Georgetown University School of Medicine, Washington, D.C.

Pachida Lo, M.D.
PGY-4 Resident, Department of Psychiatry and Behavioral Medicine, University of California, Davis, Davis, California

Linda Nahulu, M.D.
Psychiatrist, Counseling and Student Development Center, University of Hawai'i at Mānoa, Honolulu, Hawaii

Madeline Nykamp
Medical student, Creighton University School of Medicine, Omaha, Nebraska

Carine Nzodom, M.D.
PGY-4 Resident, Department of Psychiatry, School of Medicine, Louisiana State University Health, Shreveport, Louisiana

Siddarth Puri, M.D.
Child and Adolescent Psychiatry Fellow, Department of Psychiatry, University of California at Los Angeles Semel Institute for Neuroscience and Human Behavior, Los Angeles, California

Rebecca Radue, M.D.
Psychiatry Resident, Department of Psychiatry, University of Wisconsin Hospitals and Clinics, Madison, Wisconsin

Elspeth Cameron Ritchie, M.D., M.P.H., COL (retired)
Chief, Mental Health, Community Based Outpatient Clinics, Washington DC VA Medical Center; Clinical Professor of Psychiatry, George Washington University School of Medicine; Professor of Psychiatry, Howard University College of Medicine; Clinical Professor of Psychiatry, Georgetown University School of Medicine, Washington, DC; Professor of Psychiatry, Uniformed Services University of the Health Sciences, Silver Spring, Maryland

Mary Hasbah Roessel, M.D.
Adjunct Faculty, Department of Psychiatry, University of New Mexico School of Medicine; Staff Psychiatrist, Santa Fe Indian Hospital, Santa Fe, New Mexico

Samra Sahlu, M.D.
PGY-4 Resident, Department of Psychiatry, College of Medicine, University of Saskatchewan, Saskatoon, Saskatchewan, Canada

Ken Sakauye, M.D.
Emeritus Professor of Psychiatry, University of Tennessee College of Medicine, Memphis, Tennessee

Susan K. Schultz, M.D., DFAPA
Geriatric Psychiatrist, Geriatric Psychiatry, James A. Haley Veterans Hospital, Tampa, Florida; Adjunct Professor of Psychiatry, University of Iowa Carver College of Medicine, Iowa City, Iowa; Professor of Psychiatry and Behavioral Neurosciences, University of South Florida, Tampa, Florida

Daniel D. Sewell, M.D.
Professor of Clinical Psychiatry, University of California, San Diego, San Diego, California

Raissa Tanqueco, M.D.
Resident, Department of Psychiatry, University of Hawai'i at Mānoa, Honolulu, Hawaii

Nhi-Ha Trinh, M.D., M.P.H.
Assistant Professor of Psychiatry, Harvard Medical School; Director, MGH Department of Psychiatry Center for Diversity; Director of Multicultural Studies and Director of Clinical Services, MGH Depression Clinical and Research Program; Associate Director, HMS Holmes Society, Massachusetts General Hospital, Boston, Massachusetts

Lan Chi Vo, M.D.
Clinical Fellow Physician, Division of Child and Adolescent Psychiatry, Icahn School of Medicine at Mount Sinai Hospital; Resident on the Council, American Academy of Child and Adolescent Psychiatry; Psychiatry Patient Registry Online (PsychPRO) Registry Team, American Psychiatry Association, New York, New York

Mira Zein, M.D., M.P.H.
PGY-3 Resident, NYU Langone Medical Center, New York, New York

DISCLOSURE OF INTERESTS

The following contributors to this book have indicated a financial interest in or other affiliation with a commercial supporter, a manufacturer of a commercial product, a provider of a commercial service, a nongovernmental organization, and/or a government agency, as listed below:

Ebony Dix, M.D.   *Travel support:* American Psychiatric Association Leadership Fellowship to attend APA Annual Meetings and APA Components Meetings

Daniel Sewell, M.D.   *Financial:* Medical Advisory Board, ActivCare Living–Residential Memory Care, Inc. *Research support:* Higi SH, DHHS/HRSA Geriatric Workforce Enhancement Program Award

The following contributors have indicated that they have no financial interests or other affiliations that represent or could appear to represent a competing interest with the contributions to this book:

Iqbal Ahmed, M.D., FRCPsych; R. Dakota Carter, M.D.; Carl I. Cohen, M.D.; Amy Gajaria, M.D., FRCPC; Jai C. Gandhi, M.D.; Rita Hargrave, M.D.; Shuo Sally He, M.D., M.P.H.; Vicenzio Holder-Perkins, M.D., M.P.H.; Marilyn Horvath, M.D.; Raya Elfadel Kheirbek, M.D., M.P.H.; Shiv Lamba; Pachida Lo, M.D.; Maria D. Llorente, M.D., FAPA; Linda Nahulu, M.D.; Madeline Nykamp; Carine Nzodom, M.D.; Siddarth Puri, M.D.; Rebecca Radue, M.D.; Mary Hasbah Roessel, M.D.; Samra Sahlu, M.D.; Ken Sakauye, M.D.; Susan K. Schultz, M.D., DFAPA; Raissa Tanqueco, M.D.; Nhi-Ha Trinh, M.D. M.P.H.; Mira Zein, M.D., M.P.H.

Foreword

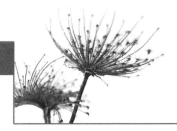

According to the U.S. Census Bureau, the year 2035 will mark an important demographic turning point in the history of the United States (Colby and Ortman 2015). For the first time ever, older adults will outnumber children. Another major demographic change relates to race and ethnicity. In 1965, 85% of the U.S. population was white. By 2050, the various racial and ethnic minorities will collectively represent a majority of the U.S. population. The older American population is also becoming racially and ethnically more diverse. Today, 78% of Americans older than age 65 are white. That proportion will drop to 57% by 2060. From 2015 to 2060, the number of black older adults in the United States will nearly triple, and that of older Hispanics or Latinos and Latinas (hereafter referred to as Latinos) will more than quadruple, whereas the number of older white adults will less than double. More racial and ethnic minority older adults live in poverty and receive worse health care compared with older whites. Similarly, there are estimated to be between 1.4 and 3.8 million lesbian, gay, bisexual, and transgender (LGBT) Americans older than age 65 (Teaster et al. 2016). With aging of the Baby Boomers, this population will increase to 3.6–7.2 million by 2030. Social isolation and discrimination experienced by many LGBT older adults hinder them from aging successfully.

These major changes in the composition of the U.S. population are bound to impact the cultural configuration of the United States. *Culture* refers to social behaviors and norms in societies and is not restricted to race and ethnicity alone. Other principles of social organization leading to cultural differences include population density (urban vs. rural), exceptional longevity (centenarians), and unique occupational exposures and experiences (e.g., military veterans). Culture is an essential factor in mental health, and it affects mental health care. Therefore, there is a critical need for a comprehensive and scholarly discussion of culture and diversity in geriatric psychiatry. This book fills that void exceedingly well. We feel honored to write the foreword for *Culture, Heritage, and Diversity in Older Adult Mental Health Care*. This topic area is fast becoming one of growing public health significance, warranting expansion of clinical care, research, and training in mental health and mental health care for various diverse groups.

Dr. Maria Llorente, a renowned authority in the field, has expertly edited the present volume, which includes outstanding contributions by a number of experts in related areas such as cultural competence, different racial and ethnic minority groups of older adults, LGBT seniors, rural elderly, centenarians, and older military veterans.

The issue of mental illness and mental health in racial and ethnic and other minorities is a complex one. Psychiatric researchers at the University of California, San Diego have focused their attention on Latinos, especially older ones, during the past several years. Below we consider a few salient aspects of culture and diversity as they apply to this group, to illustrate the impact of culture on mental health care. Various other minority groups face somewhat similar and somewhat different concerns and considerations.

It is important to note that there is significant diversity within Latinos in the United States. Latinos vary in country of origin or descent, language use, race, and immigration history (Marquine et al. 2015b). These variations between and within Latino subgroups may impact mental health outcomes and their predictors. At the same time, it is also necessary to recognize that most Latinos share a number of salient experiences in a more or less prominent way in their personal history or heritage, including the Spanish language and the immigrant experience. There are also certain cultural values that tend to permeate the lives of Latinos, such as familism (key role of the family) and collectivism (importance of the group rather than the individual).

The reported prevalence of mental illnesses among Latinos is variable. However, several studies have found lower rates of psychiatric disorders in Latino immigrants than in non-Latino whites, despite lower socioeconomic status. Identification of psychobiosocial strengths in Latinos that are associated with this so-called "Hispanic paradox" of mental health could provide key insights for Latinos' mental health. Consistent with this notion, we have found that community-based older Latinos living in San Diego county reported increased satisfaction with life compared with a demographically matched non-Latino white group. Furthermore, higher spirituality among Latinos was an important factor explaining this difference (Marquine et al. 2015a).

Acculturation is the process by which individuals adopt the attitudes, values, customs, beliefs, and behaviors of another culture. Language has consistently been the most frequently used proxy for, and strongest measure of, acculturation in Latinos. One of our studies involved large numbers of Spanish-speaking Latinos, English-speaking Latinos, and non-Latino whites initiating treatment for schizophrenia, bipolar disorder, or major depression (Folsom et al. 2007). We found that compared with English-speaking Latinos and non-Latino whites, Spanish-speaking Latinos were less likely to enter care through emergency or jail services and more likely to enter care through outpatient services. Thus, for Latinos, preferred language, or degree of acculturation into the mainstream culture, may be more important than self-reported ethnicity alone in mental health service use.

Psychotropic medication nonadherence is a major public health problem. A systematic review of the literature showed that rates of nonadherence to psychotropic medications were significantly higher for Latinos than for non-Latino whites (Lanouette et al. 2009). This has important clinical implications for psychopharmacological treatment of Latinos.

The prevalence of dementia among U.S. Latinos is expected to increase sixfold by 2050 as this segment of the population ages. Yet there is a serious lack of availability of culturally and linguistically appropriate health care services such as neurocognitive testing for older Latinos. This issue is exacerbated for rural Latino populations, who have even worse access to and utilization of health care services. Therefore, culturally acceptable and easily administered interventions designed for this specific population can have a significant impact. In one study, we found that neurocognitive assessment via telepsychiatry using a Spanish-language battery was comparable to in-person testing using the same battery in Spanish-speaking older adults in a rural setting (Vahia et al. 2015). Like telemedicine, telepsychiatry can be of considerable value for older Latinos with cognitive impairment.

There is also a critical need for developing and testing culturally sensitive interventions for serious mental illnesses in diverse groups. In a study of Latinos with persistent psychotic disorders, Mausbach et al. (2008) reported that a culturally tailored skills training intervention resulted in significant improvement in performance-based skills assessment and well-being compared with a nontailored intervention. These results indicate that Latinos with serious mental illnesses can benefit from interventions that consider cultural values and mores.

Another problematic issue is a widening disparity between the proportion of ethnic minority Americans in the population and the number of researchers from these minority groups. Although blacks, Latinos, and American Indians compose 26% of the U.S. population, they receive only 16% of the undergraduate degrees and 9% of the doctorate degrees in science and engineering. Likewise, whereas 10% of National Institutes of Health (NIH) trainees are members of these ethnic minority groups, they make up only 3%–4% of the principal investigators on NIH- and National Institute of Mental health–funded research and program grants. One of the most critical ingredients for the development of a research career is the mentor, yet current academic settings present serious barriers to the creation and sustenance of a mentor workforce. A focus on recruitment, training, and retention of mentors for underrepresented minority trainees is clearly warranted (Jeste et al. 2009).

To conclude, there is an urgent need to study older people from various minority groups and to develop effective interventions that are culturally sensitive. This book is an excellent step in that direction. We want to compliment the editor and the authors of the chapters of this remarkable book for publishing a timely, insightful, and thought-provoking volume that should be of great interest to anyone interested in the broad of topics of mental health, culture, and aging.

Dilip V. Jeste, M.D.

Departments of Psychiatry and Neurosciences, Sam and Rose Stein Institute for Research on Aging, University of California San Diego, San Diego, California

María J. Marquine, Ph.D.

Departments of Psychiatry and Neurosciences, Sam and Rose Stein Institute for Research on Aging, University of California San Diego, San Diego, California

REFERENCES

Colby SL, Ortman JM: U.S. Census Bureau Projections of the Size and Composition of the U.S. Population: 2014 to 2060: Population Estimates and Projections. Suitland, MD, U.S. Census Bureau, 2015

Folsom DP, Gilmer T, Barrio C, et al: A longitudinal study of the use of mental health services by persons with serious mental illness: do Spanish-speaking Latinos differ from English-speaking Latinos and Caucasians? Am J Psychiatry 164(8):1173–1180, 2007 17671279

Jeste DV, Twamley EW, Cardenas V, et al: A call for training the trainers: focus on mentoring to enhance diversity in mental health research. Am J Public Health 99(suppl 1):S31–S37, 2009 19246662

Lanouette NM, Folsom DP, Sciolla A, Jeste DV: Psychotropic medication non-adherence among United States Latinos: a comprehensive literature review. Psychiatr Serv 60(2):157–174, 2009 19176409

Marquine MJ, Maldonado Y, Zlatar Z, et al: Differences in life satisfaction among older community-dwelling Hispanics and non-Hispanic whites. Aging Ment Health 19(11):978–988, 2015a 25402813

Marquine MJ, Zlatar ZZ, Sewell DD: Positive geriatric and cultural psychiatry, in Positive Psychiatry: A Clinical Handbook. Edited by Jeste DV, Palmer BW. Arlington, VA, American Psychiatric Publishing, 2015b, pp 305–323

Mausbach BT, Budardo J, McKibbin CL, et al: Evaluation of a culturally tailored skills intervention for Latinos with persistent psychotic disorders. Am J Psychiatr Rehabil 11(1):61–75, 2008 19779589

Teaster PB, White JT, Kim S: Sexual minority status and aging, in Handbook of LGBT Elders. Edited by Harley DA, Teaster PB. Cham, Switzerland, Springer International, 2016, pp 27–42

Vahia IV, Ng B, Camacho A, et al: Telepsychiatry for neurocognitive testing in older rural Latino adults. Am J Geriatric Psychiatry 23(7):666–670, 2015 25708655

Preface

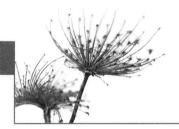

Se formo un arroz con mango. It formed a rice with mango. To Cubans, Venezuelans, and others from Central America, the meaning of this expression is clear: a big mess, a complication, a confusion occurred. To other Latinos, however, this expression has no significance, and it clearly loses something in the translation. That is the essence of understanding diversity and culture: what is clear to one group forms *arroz con mango* in another. Nowhere is this understanding more critically important than when dealing with the mental health care of older adults. In this book, we seek to enhance the understanding of health care providers and trainees regarding the diversity of current and future seniors.

In May 2016, at the Annual Meeting of the American Psychiatric Association (APA), one of the members of the Council on Geriatric Psychiatry described difficulty finding resource materials to use in training her residents and fellows about cultural sensitivity and competency with respect to minority elderly who came to their clinical settings. She was directed to the Cultural Competency Curriculum that had been developed by the Ethnic Minority Elderly (EME) Subcommittee of the APA Council on Aging, we thought just a few years before. When we sought the link to the online curriculum, we discovered that the work had been completed 10 years before. There was consensus among council members that an update was needed because there was now a much larger body of literature.

As the committee discussed the proposed scope, it became clear that the greatest value added would be to include the original major ethnic and racial groups (African American, Latino, Asian and Pacific Islander, and Indigenous peoples) and add other groups that were not initially included: underserved populations (rural elderly) and diverse specialty groups (lesbian, gay, bisexual, and transgender individuals; veterans; and centenarians). This expansion reflected the increasing diversity of the aging population and the recognition that persons from these specialty groups have unique life experiences and occupational exposures that increase the risk for certain types of psychiatric disorders in later life.

Each chapter has a senior author and, in most cases, junior faculty and trainees as authors. The senior author is a recognized subject matter expert on the given group of seniors. The junior authors participated in literature searches and reviews as well as manuscript writing. This group is diverse and includes representatives of each of the groups discussed in the book, except centenarians. Levels of training included a high school student, a medical student, several psychiatry residents, several geriatric psychiatry fellows, APA fellows, and junior faculty.

The first three chapters provide overviews; training techniques; and the concepts of cultural competence, adaptation, acculturation, and assimilation and discuss how these aspects interact with psychiatric conditions. The group-specific chapters summarize the literature regarding that group of seniors, including demographics, prevalence of psychiatric disorders, presentation and treatment considerations, and group-specific specialty information.

This work would not have been possible without the volunteer time of the authors. I thank each one profusely for their willingness to participate, meeting timelines and producing an exceptional body of knowledge that cannot be found elsewhere. Their work fosters understanding and communication that ultimately will improve the mental health care delivered to older adults.

I am also extremely grateful to Ike Ahmed, who chaired the EME Subcommittee and edited the original Cultural Competency Curriculum. Ike offered guidance, wisdom, and sage advice. He is a consummate teacher and mentor, involving trainees in almost every aspect of academic work, and he served as a role model, leading to the involvement of so many trainees in this book. I would like to acknowledge the original authors of that work (many of whom participated in this book), including Warachal E. Faison, Kenneth M. Sakauye, Elizabeth J. Kramer, Mia J. Robinson, Nhi-Ha T. Trinh, Yolonda R. Colemon, and Cynthia I. Resendez.

I would also like to thank Dr. Robert Roca, the Chair of the Council on Geriatric Psychiatry, and Dr. Ranna Parekh, Director of the APA Division of Diversity and Health Equity, whose tireless support and advocacy were instrumental in making this publication possible. Finally, I would like to thank Sejal Patel, who facilitated communication among and between the authors and connected us with other APA offices, staff, committees, and resources.

Our hope is that this work will prevent the formation of *arroz con mango* and that it will enhance your work with older adults. After all, sooner or later, we will be those older adults or those who care for them. Maya Angelou said it best in *Wouldn't Take Nothing for My Journey Now*: "…by demonstrating that all peoples cry, laugh, eat, worry and die, it can introduce the idea that if we try and understand each other, we may even become friends."

Maria D. Llorente, M.D., FAPA

CHAPTER 1

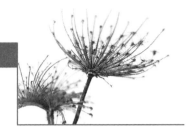

Why Is Cultural Competency Important When Working With Older Adults?

Amy Gajaria, M.D., FRCPC
Ebony Dix, M.D.
Ken Sakauye, M.D.
Maria D. Llorente, M.D., FAPA

Learning Objectives

Become familiar with the demographic transformation currently under way in the United States, where the population is getting older and becoming increasingly more diverse.

Understand the importance and benefits of establishing a culturally competent health care system.

Appreciate the unique role of communication, in various formats, in obtaining a history and establishing a treatment plan for older adults from diverse backgrounds.

Become acquainted with evidence-based models of culturally competent health care services delivery.

Recognize how principles of the scientific method can be used to facilitate discussions regarding the experience of prejudice and discrimination.

DEMOGRAPHICS

In the United States, the population is expanding and getting older, as it is throughout the world (Ortman et al. 2014). However, the older adult population in the United States is also becoming increasingly diverse. This is due to trends in international migration, mortality, and childbearing. By 2050, the overall Hispanic population in the United States will increase to 103 million, nearly doubling in size from 13% to 24% of the total U.S. population; in older adults, Hispanics make up 20% of those older than 65 years (Seltzer and Yahirun 2013). Similarly, the proportion of Asians in the United States is projected to triple, from 11 million to 33 million, representing a growth to 8% of the total population. The African American population is projected to grow from 36 million to 61 million, an increase of 71%, which will represent 15% of the total U.S. population by 2050 (U.S. Census Bureau 2015; Vincent and Velkoff 2010). By 2050, projections indicate that 35% of the population older than 65 will be from a racial or ethnic minority group—compared with 11% in 1970. The largest growth rates are predicted to be among Hispanics, African Americans, Asian and Pacific Islanders, and American Indians (Lehman et al. 2012).

Racial and ethnic minorities disproportionately interact with the health care system because they are more likely to have higher prevalence of chronic diseases. Compared with non-Hispanic whites, African Americans and Latinos are more likely to have at least one of the following illnesses: diabetes, cardiovascular disease, hypertension, obesity, asthma, cancer, or anxiety/depression (Georgetown University Health Policy Institute 2004). Health care providers and organizations need to deliver services that meet the social, cultural, and linguistic needs of the patients they serve. By delivering this culturally competent care, systems can improve health outcomes and quality of care, as well as reduce or eliminate health care disparities. To achieve these goals, health care professionals must receive training on cultural competence in order to develop and establish systems of care that reduce access barriers, deliver true patient-centered care, and enhance health care outcomes.

DEFINITIONS OF CULTURE AND CULTURALLY COMPETENT CARE

The term *culture* is multifaceted and may refer to one's belief system, values, religion, race, socioeconomic status, ethnicity, language, sexual orientation, geographic location, educational level, age, occupational risks and exposures, and gender. *Cultural competence* in health care systems is defined as the ability to understand and integrate these features into the provision of health care services. Brach and Fraser (2000) listed common strategies for delivering culturally competent care, including interpreter services; hiring minority staff who reflect the population served; training to increase cultural awareness, knowledge, and skills; inclusion of traditional healers; use of community health workers; incorporation of culture-specific attitudes and values throughout the health care system; involvement of family in health care decision making; geographically accessible clinics; flexible hours of operation; and linguistic competency in both administrative and clinical encounters.

Culturally competent care has been described by the National Quality Forum (NQF; Weech-Maldonado et al. 2012a, 2012b) as "the ongoing capacity of health care systems, organizations, and professionals to provide for diverse patient populations high-quality care that is safe, patient and family centered, evidence based, and equitable" (Weech-Maldonado et al. 2012a, p. 55). This entails ongoing engagement by health care professionals in developing a heightened awareness and understanding of the patient within his or her cultural context. Additionally, the NQF describes how organizations must develop a comprehensive framework inclusive of both management and clinical subsystems in order to meet the needs of a diverse workforce and patient population (National Quality Forum 2009). The framework consists of six total domains, four of which are management related—leadership, integration into management systems and operations, workforce delivery and training, and community engagement—and two of which are clinically related—patient-provider communication and mechanisms that support care delivery (Weech-Maldonado et al. 2012a).

CULTURAL COMPETENCE AND HEALTH CARE OUTCOMES

The significance of cultural competence within health care organizations has been echoed not only by the promulgation of federal laws and regulations, as well as regulations by accreditation bodies, but also by the multitude of research and data published regarding this topic. Research data indicate that a lack of culturally competent care leads to poor patient outcomes, poor adherence, and an increase in health disparities (Lehman et al. 2012). For example, heart failure in African Americans illustrates how diagnostic and treatment decisions regarding certain diseases are often influenced by a patient's ethnicity or racial background (Dries et al. 1999). There is a higher prevalence of heart failure and cardiovascular disease in the African American population, in part due to differences in genetic polymorphisms. However, it has been well established in the medical literature that socioeconomic factors and quality of care contribute largely to the disparity associated with treatment outcomes in African Americans versus whites (Wierenga et al. 2016). A study conducted by the American Heart Association examined cardiovascular disease awareness among American women and found significantly lower awareness among black (31%) and Hispanic (29%) women when compared with white women (68%) (Christian et al. 2007).

Disparities in access to and quality of health care are not unique only to race, ethnicity, and gender. Minority populations also include individuals with lower socioeconomic status in the aging population. Lower-income individuals tend to have lower health care literacy, inadequate access to preventive care, delay in seeking treatment for symptoms, and nonadherence with follow-up appointments and recommended treatment (Sharma et al. 2014). Findings from the *2016 National Healthcare Disparities Report* (U.S. Department of Health and Human Services 2016) illustrate that compared with high-income individuals, poor individuals not only have barriers to access to health care but also receive suboptimal quality of care. The long-term and costly impact of these negative outcomes will be magnified as the aging population continues to grow and diversify. Further, the Institute of Medicine (2003) reported that for racial and ethnic populations, the lack of culturally and linguistically competent providers further compounds the problem.

Systematic reviews of the medical literature have examined studies designed to train health professionals to improve cultural competence, and all have shown an overall improvement in attitudes and skills of health professionals as well as patient satisfaction (Beach et al. 2005; Truong et al. 2014). Weech-Maldonado et al. (2012b) examined the relationship between cultural competency and patients' experience within the inpatient setting by using the Cultural Competency Assessment Tool for Hospitals (CCATH) and found a positive relationship between hospital cultural competence and patient experiences with care. The Centers for Medicare and Medicaid Services use a standardized survey called the Hospital Consumer Assessment of Healthcare Providers and Systems (HCAHPS) to collect data on patient experiences with care. This allows for quality improvement initiatives to be implemented in health care systems, which can produce measurable results in the form of higher HCAHPS scores.

Reducing health care disparities not only improves population health outcomes but also impacts cost and the overall economics of health care (Villablanca et al. 2016). Health care organizations are now recognizing the importance of cultural competence as it relates to efficiency, quality, and equity in the delivery of care within a competitive health care market. This can also incentivize the health care organizations that accept Medicare and Medicaid to implement standards that comply with those regulations and purchasing practices (Brach and Fraser 2002). Some other benefits to an organization of providing culturally competent health care include improvement in cost-effectiveness in caring for patients, an increase in market share by appealing to minority consumers, and overall performance improvement. An increase in performance on quality measures may be of particular interest to private purchasers, particularly in competitive markets with a large minority population (Butler et al. 2016).

Additionally, a health care organization's policies and practices regarding cultural competency facilitate internal communications among the workforce, reducing disparities in career outcomes and enhancing organizational performance (Meyers 2007). Key components of the development and implementation of a culturally competent framework within a health care system include organizational, structural, and clinical cultural competence (Betancourt et al. 2002). On the basis of this concept, Weech-Maldonado et al. (2016) conducted a study that examined the impact of a systematic cultural competency initiative on specific hospital performance metrics. Their results showed improvements in organizational outcomes as a result of honing in on competencies that were at both an organizational and an individual level. Organizational-level competencies that were taught included diversity leadership, strategic human resource management, and patient cultural competency. Individual-level domains included attitudes toward diversity, recognition of implicit biases, and understanding racial or ethnic identities. The results suggested that an effective strategy in the development of culturally competent care in a health care organization involves a holistic approach.

LANGUAGE AND CULTURAL COMPETENCE

Linguistic competence, defined broadly as effective communication with persons speaking a nondominant language, is an essential component of culturally competent health care, and it is of particular importance in mental health care. The inability of patients to communicate effectively with their health care provider has been identified as a barrier to quality access to health care not only by patients (Anderson et al. 2003; Tucker et al. 2003) but also by both providers and governing bodies (Brach and Fraser 2002; Renzaho et al. 2013). Patients report that being unable to communicate effectively with their health care provider causes them increased distress, results in feeling misunderstood, increases distrust in the medical system, and decreases their willingness to access health care (Anderson et al. 2003). When providers attempt to address communication barriers by using simple language, patients report feeling that the provider sees them as "stupid" or "uneducated," which decreases patients' willingness to seek care (Pollack et al. 2012; Quach et al. 2012). In addition, difficulties in communication can affect a practitioner's ability to provide an accurate diagnosis and can affect a practitioner's ability to provide appropriate medical and psychiatric care (Betancourt et al. 2003; U.S. Department of Health and Human Services 2001).

Communication in this context refers not only to direct verbal communication between patient and provider but also written health information, signage within clinics, ability to interpret nonverbal or emotional cues, and verbal communication with nonprovider staff (e.g., staff responsible for scheduling or billing, telephone operators) patients may encounter while accessing health care. With respect to direct communication between patient and provider, the gold standard is a provider who is fluent in the patient's language and is familiar with medical terminology within that language. This has the benefit of maintaining patient confidentiality, promoting a sense of trust and understanding between patient and provider, and increasing overall trust in the health system where the provider works by increasing diversity within this particular health care setting (U.S. Department of Health and Human Services 2001). However, this is not possible in many situations, particularly in multiethnic settings where multiple different languages are spoken by patients.

The next best option for appropriate communication is to use a trained medical interpreter (Kirmayer 2012; U.S. Department of Health and Human Services 2001). Interpreters should be bilingual in the dominant language as well as the language of the patient and should be comfortable with using medical language to effectively translate material between patient and provider (Kirmayer et al. 2011; U.S. Department of Health and Human Services 2001). Providers should have an understanding of the interpretation services available in their treatment setting and should have the skills to communicate effectively through an interpreter.

In some situations, patients may request to not have in-person interpretation because their linguistic community is small and they feel that in-person interpretation might not maintain their confidentiality. This is particularly true when a patient presents with mental health concerns. In addition, there may be emergency situations when it is not possible to wait to obtain the services of an in-person interpreter. In these situations, it may be more suitable to use telephone interpretation services; however, these services should not be considered a substitute for in-person interpretation in nonemergency settings.

Family and friends, particularly children of older patients, should not be used to interpret medical information unless explicitly requested by the patient. Family and friends may not have the level of fluency, particularly in relation to medical terminology, to interpret medical information effectively, and they may not have the ability to directly and accurately communicate information between patient and provider. In addition, informal interpretation provides a false sense of security between provider and informal interpreter in which the provider assumes the informal interpreter is interpreting information in the same manner that a trained interpreter might. Informal interpretation, whether by family, friends, or nonfluent medical staff, has resulted in problematic communication in health care settings (Betancourt et al. 2003; U.S. Department of Health and Human Services 2001). In situations when the patient requests that a family member provide interpretation, the patient should be informed that interpretation must be made available to him or her at no cost as mandated by law in the United States (U.S. Department of Health and Human Services 2001).

Even with the use of a trained interpreter, this form of communication poses challenges in mental health settings, where conveying empathy and understanding nonverbal cues are essential to developing rapport and establishing an appropriate diagnosis (Bhui et al. 2007). In addition, it can be difficult to discern information about a patient's thought processes when an interview is conducted through an interpreter. This can be particularly challenging when attempting to evaluate the presence of a psychotic disorder. In mental health settings, providers can request that the interpreter comment on the nature of the language spoken in order to inform the mental status examination and can request that the interpreter interpret language as closely as possible to obtain a more accurate understanding of the patient's thought process (Kirmayer et al. 2011), which can help to address some of these challenges.

At the same time, patients are also attentive to the physician's nonverbal communication and have reported feeling that physicians and health care institutions can communicate irritation or frustration when having to accommodate language barriers (Pollack et al. 2012). Even patients who speak English as a first language, including second-generation Hispanics and African Americans, report feeling that they are misunderstood or that they have to change their way of speaking to feel comfortable in health care settings, suggesting that more attention needs to be paid to nonverbal communication in cross-cultural and cross-linguistic settings (Johnson et al. 2004).

Communication in health care settings also often involves written materials and signage. These environmental aspects of care are sometimes forgotten when considering how to provide effective cross-cultural care, and if patients cannot effectively navigate these materials, this adds another barrier to care (Nyblade et al. 2009). Written communication, although not a substitute for medical interpretation, can help ensure that patients understand essential aspects of their care, including the nature of their diagnosis; recommended treatment options; how to take medication as prescribed; common side effects; and how to navigate through a hospital or clinic setting, particularly with older adults who may experience mobility difficulties.

Finally, patients report that interactions with nonmedical health care staff can have a significant impact on how they experience their treatment, informing how likely they are to access care. For example, front desk clerical staff are often the first encounter the patient has with the health care system. Difficulties booking appointments or communicating with the staff due to language barriers can result in barriers to mental health access. This may be exacerbated in the case of older adults who may have the added difficulty of poor hearing. Patients report that they make decisions on whether to access services on the basis of prior experiences with a treatment setting, and a prior bad experience, whether related to their interaction with a care provider or to nonmedical clinic staff, can decrease their willingness to access care again (Anderson et al. 2003; Pollack et al. 2012).

Ensuring effective cross-linguistic communication is not easy and requires attention to many factors outside direct verbal communication between patient and provider. However, the alternative—in which non-English-speaking patients receive ineffective medical care and providers are at risk for making incorrect diagnoses and thus offering improper treatments—can have serious (if not life-threatening) consequences not only for the health of older adults with mental health difficulties but also for the providers and institutions that wish to effectively care for them in compassionate and welcoming settings.

Designs of Health Care Systems That Are Culturally Competent

Models of culturally competent health care organizations have been emerging across the country for several decades, especially with the advent of national policies and guidelines set forth by various entities. These guidelines and policies give different organizations the necessary tools by which to improve performance, train and educate staff, and help inform policy. The U.S. Department of Health and Human Resources has played an integral role in establishing and implementing standards of culturally competent care through its various divisions. The Agency for Healthcare Research and Quality works within the department to improve the safety and quality of the health care system through research. In 2001, another division, the Office of Minority Health, published national standards for Culturally and Linguistically Appropriate Services (CLAS) in health care, giving organizations standards to which to adhere (U.S. Department of Health and Human Services 2001). CCATH was eventually developed as a tool to assess adherence to the CLAS standards. Other examples include the NQF's publication of *A Comprehensive Framework and Preferred Practices for Measuring and Reporting Cultural Competency* in 2008 (National Quality Forum 2009) and The Joint Commission's publication of *Advancing Effective Communication, Cultural Competence, and Patient- and Family-Centered Care: A Roadmap for Hospitals* in 2010 (The Joint Commission 2010).

White Memorial Medical Center (WMMC) in Los Angeles, California developed a Family Practice Residency Program in the late 1980s with a mission to serve the local community, which was predominantly Mexican American (Betancourt et al. 2002). The center created a cross-cultural curriculum in the 1990s that specifically devoted time to cultural competency training for residents and faculty. This included case presentations with an emphasis on sociocultural perspectives and a faculty retreat that helped to integrate cultural competence into all teaching at WMMC. With continued support from The California Endowment, the WMMC has developed the Cultural Competence Initiative for Physician Training Programs. The focus of the program is to educate physicians on the values, beliefs, practices, and communication needs of the diverse Hispanic patient population in East Lost Angeles.

The Washington State Department of Social and Health Services launched a program for immigrants with limited English proficiency in 1991 in response to several lawsuits and civil rights complaints regarding unequal access to services by consumers with limited English proficiency (LEP). The program, which was initially called Language Interpreter Services and Translations, provided training for interpreters and translators and offered translation assistance to LEP consumers at no cost (Betancourt et al. 2002). Today, it is called the Language Testing and Certification program. The program has been revised and amended over the years but continues to provide services to LEP populations within the state.

Kaiser Permanente in San Francisco, California, is an example of a managed care organization that has developed a system of culturally competent care on a national level. In the 1990s, in response to studies that indicated high rates of dissatisfaction with Kaiser Permanente's delivery of health care within the Asian population in Northern California, the organization developed an initiative to find a solution to remedy this issue. As a result of this community health initiative, Kaiser Permanente established a department of multicultural services that provides on-site interpretation services in 14 different languages and dialects (Betancourt et al. 2002). The organization also developed a translation unit responsible for translating appropriate signage and written materials and a cultural advisory board to oversee the department. Kaiser later developed modules of culturally targeted health care delivery to include Latino patients, which have expanded to multiple centers targeting other minority groups. Currently, there are centers that focus on other minority groups such as African Americans, Eastern European populations, individuals with disabilities, and women.

Sunset Park Family Health Center Network of Lutheran Medical Center, located in Sunset Park, Brooklyn, an underserved neighborhood in New York City, was developed in the 1960s as a community health center aimed at delivering culturally competent health care to its ethnically diverse and impoverished population. Inhabitants of this neighborhood include populations from Scandinavia, Puerto Rico, Central and South America, Russia, and Middle Eastern countries. In response to the need for primary care in this ethnically diverse area, the center developed initiatives that focused on particular groups, such the Asian Initiative and later the Mexican Initiative (Betancourt et al. 2002). These initiatives aimed at reducing barriers to care and eventually formed the foundation for what is today a community-based health care system that celebrates diversity. Celebrating various religious and cultural holidays, displaying multicultural artwork, offering a variety of ethnic foods, and creating a nondenominational prayer room on site are examples of how a culturally competent infrastructure may be created at the community level and expanded statewide (Betancourt et al. 2002). In addition, the organization has expanded to include training programs for staff, patient navigators, and community outreach workers. It eventually partnered with the Lutheran Medical Center of New York University (now NYU Langone Hospital—Brooklyn), and currently, there are several affiliated sites throughout New York State that provide medical, behavioral health, and dental care.

Campinha-Bacote (2002), an advocate and consultant on transcultural health care and mental health nursing, developed the Culturally

Competent Model of Care, which encompasses five main constructs related to the key components of care. These constructs are as follows
(Lehman et al. 2012):

1. *Cultural awareness*—a self-reflection of one's own biases
2. *Cultural knowledge*—obtaining information about different cultures
3. *Cultural skill*—conducting an assessment of cultural data of the patient
4. *Cultural encounters*—personal experiences with patients of different
   backgrounds
5. *Cultural desire*—the process of wanting to be culturally competent

Regardless of the specific sector—academia, government, managed
care, community health—the aforementioned designs of these culturally competent health care systems (White Memorial, Washington State,
Kaiser Permanente, and Sunset Park) share a similar framework. This
framework comprises key components that are essential to the development and implementation of effective, culturally competent health care.
These components take into account verbal and nonverbal communication, sociocultural influences on patients' beliefs and behaviors, understanding how these influences can cause barriers to access, and ability
to devise strategies to reduce disparities.

CULTURALLY COMPETENT DISCUSSIONS REGARDING PREJUDICE AND DISCRIMINATION

Prejudice is defined as a preconceived notion ("prejudging") that typically has no basis in fact and often forms a negative attitude toward
members of a particular group of people. The groups could be based on
such factors as gender, race, age, geography, nationality, sexual orientation, religion, political opinions, educational or socioeconomic level, or
occupation. *Discrimination*, on the other hand, is the recognition and understanding of the difference between one thing or person and another.
It is not inherently problematic. Each day, we discriminate between
foods we prefer to eat or choices that are right or wrong. It is when one
engages in the unjust or prejudicial treatment of specific categories of
people that discrimination becomes problematic. Some have suggested
that prejudice is internal thoughts and feelings and discrimination is the
translation of those thoughts and feelings into action. The remainder of
this chapter will focus on the problematic aspects of discrimination.

The experience of discrimination is an unfortunately common experience for many different groups of people. For example, in one study, 25% of African Americans reported at least one experience of discrimination in the previous year (McLaughlin et al. 2010). This discrimination can occur in the workplace, school, or personal settings and is often driven largely by unconscious biases, of which the individual is at times unaware. As with transference and countertransference, mental health practitioners and patients do not need to correct their unconscious biases unless these biases have harmful effects on their decisions and interactions with others. However, in the case of race and ethnicity, addressing prejudice and its effects is more than political correctness; it is a prerequisite to delivering high-quality health care services.

These biases can take many forms. The patient has biases about the cause of his or her medical illness, type of treatment that should be given, or trustworthiness of the doctor or the health care system. The doctor may have biases about the patient based on his or her age, race, ethnicity, nationality, gender, socioeconomic status, education, sexual orientation, and even use of language and grammar.

A major problem with these unconscious biases is that no one thinks he or she is prejudiced or biased, and people tend to apply confirmation bias while giving disproportionately less consideration to alternative possibilities. Psychiatry has tried to curb acting on bias through the application of the scientific method to the clinical interview (Table 1–1) and suspension of judgment until enough information is present that the practitioner can be relatively confident of his or her formulation. Applied in the everyday clinical encounter, use of the scientific method, using qualitative methods with all patients, leads to a culturally competent assessment.

Before the scientific method was applied in clinical psychiatry (Kendler 1990), unverified assumptions led to underuse of formal mental health services. These practices failed to include patient-preferred alternative care such as family or spiritual involvement, including rituals and herbal remedies, or lacked insight into cultural beliefs, such as thinking a given illness is a "normal" part of aging. Underuse and low access are often due to the inherent fear of mistreatment by a system that the patient does not trust. Evidence suggests that people who experience discrimination outside the health care setting, particularly when such experiences are felt to be supported by larger institutional structures, are less likely to access health care for the fear that they will again face discrimination (Anderson et al. 2003; Hall et al. 2015; Quach et al. 2012). Reports of individuals who describe explicit and implicit experiences of discrimination within the health care setting, including

TABLE 1–1. Example of application of the scientific method to cultural issues

Step	Application
Determine the question to be answered	Why is the patient so angry with me when we have only just met?
Do background research	Obtain knowledge of the patient's ethnicity and that group's history in the United States (and, if the patient is foreign born, in country of origin). Interview the patient, asking for information on how he or she was treated when getting the appointment.
Construct a hypothesis	The patient is afraid of mistreatment or being a guinea pig.
Test the hypothesis	Review responses to queries in the interview and things the patient says.
Analyze your data and draw a conclusion	The conclusion should be based on whatever is inferred from the data.
Communicate your results	Provide your interpretation to the patient.

name-calling and racial slurs, can lead to the sense that some patients are looked down on and treated differently (in a negative way) from others (Johnson et al. 2004; Pollack et al. 2012).

Additionally, there is a robust body of evidence demonstrating that experiences of discrimination have serious effects on a person's physical and mental well-being, with some studies likening the effect to that of a chronic illness (Pascoe and Smart Richman 2009). Discrimination, particularly when it is repetitive and chronic, has significant adverse effects on the mental health of a person, ranging from decreased reports of subjective well-being to increased rates of depression and anxiety (Díaz et al. 2001; Pascoe and Smart Richman 2009). These effects persist even when controlling for other social determinants of health, including socioeconomic status, level of insurance coverage, and disease severity (Smedley et al. 2003).

Although there is evidence supporting the negative effects of discrimination on individuals, there is more limited research to guide providers in addressing these experiences on an individual patient level. Various interventions have been suggested to help practitioners care for patients who may have experienced discrimination. As with other approaches to culturally competent care, one approach is to strive for a diverse workforce, particularly one in which minority identities are visible. This approach has been shown to increase minority patients' comfort with accessing health care even in the absence of other interventions (Kirmayer et al. 2011). In addition, if institutional health care structures partner with community organizations that serve minority communities, this can signal to patients from those communities that the health care organization is interested in their needs (Nyblade et al. 2009). Such partnerships can include involving community partners in program development or in conversations about the physical infrastructure of the treatment setting (Cross et al. 1989). It can also involve providing care outside the clinic setting within the setting of a community organization or inviting community or religious organizations to provide services from within the health care setting. These partnerships are generally most effective when they are bilateral and when both organizations have an equal voice and derive benefit from the partnership.

DSM-5 now includes the Cultural Formulation Interview (CFI), which, from an individual clinical perspective, focuses on the patient's view of the illness; the patient's own attempts at treatment; the people to whom he or she turns for help; and potential barriers to treatment, including unwillingness to work with the interviewer (American Psychiatric Association 2013) (Table 1–2). This is a marked departure from DSM-IV, which viewed cultural issues as unusual culture-bound syndromes that are rare even in the cultural groups in which they occur (American Psychiatric Association 1994). Applying the CFI is the preferred method for getting information from all patients. Details and course of symptoms can be queried as the interview proceeds.

The question of how providers should address instances of discrimination with their individual patients is a more challenging one. Patients who are unable to find a place to discuss their experiences of discrimination are found to have poorer mental health outcomes than do those who do have such an outlet (McLaughlin et al. 2010), and social support can moderate the effects of discrimination on mental health (Pascoe and Smart Richman 2009). This could perhaps be addressed by ensuring that patients are aware of resources serving their community, although not all may feel they can relate to these resources.

Particularly vulnerable are those patients who may not feel connected to their community. This can happen for a number of reasons. A patient with intersecting minority identities (e.g., a patient who identifies as lesbian, gay, bisexual, transgender, or queer/questioning who is also African American) may not feel at home in organizations addressing only one of these identities and may feel even more isolated by this

---

TABLE 1–2. Cultural Formulation Interview

---

1. What brings you here today?

2. Sometimes people have different ways of describing their problem to their family, friends, or others in the community. How would describe your problem to them?

3. What troubles you most about your problem?

4. Why do you think this is happening to you? What do you think are the causes?

5. What do others in your family, your friends, or others in your community think is causing your problem?

6. Are there any kinds of support that makes your problem better, such as support from family friends, or others?

7. Are there any kinds of stresses that make your problem worse?

8. For you, what are the most important aspects of your background or identity?

9. Are there any aspects of your background or identity that make a difference to your problem?

10. Are there any aspects of your background or identity that are causing other concerns or difficulties for you?

11. Sometimes people have various ways of dealing with problems like this. What have you done on your own to cope?

12. Often people look for help from many different sources, including different kinds of doctors, helpers, or healers. In the past, what kinds of treatment, help, advice, or healing have you sought? Which were most helpful?

13. Has anything prevented you from getting the help you need?

14. What kinds of help do you think would be most useful to you at this time?

15. Are there other kinds of help that your family, friends, or other people have suggested that would be helpful for you now?

16. Sometimes doctors and patients misunderstand each other because they come from different backgrounds or have different expectations. Have you been concerned about this, and is there anything that we can do to provide you with the care you need?

Source. Adapted from American Psychiatric Association: *Diagnostic and Statistical Manual of Mental Disorders*, 5th Edition, Arlington, VA, American Psychiatric Association, 2013, pp. 752–754. Copyright © 2013 American Psychiatric Association. Used with permission.

experience. Another patient who is a second- or third-generation immigrant may find it hard to relate to community organizations that serve first-generation immigrants or newcomers. Patients may live in rural geographic areas or belong to smaller ethnic groups for whom there are no preexisting community services. Conversely, there may be a given community resource, but the individual comes from a country where a recent civil war has caused a rift between the members of that nationality, and members of the local community are potentially on opposing sides of the conflict.

A practitioner also may wish to provide a safe space to allow patients to discuss their experiences of discrimination, particularly in the context of psychotherapy or a longer-term relationship. Again, the guidelines derived from the literature are somewhat limited. The literature suggests that before providers consider having these discussions with patients, they should examine their own relationship to their individual identities and their experience of discrimination or lack thereof (American Counseling Association 1992; American Psychological Association 2003; National Association of Social Workers 2015). Those who wish to have these conversations with patients should have a space to develop a reflective practice in which they are able to address the challenging feelings that come up when discussing issues of discrimination, particularly when the provider's and patient's experiences of discrimination are discordant (American Psychological Association 2003). This can be achieved through individual self-reflection or through finding a like-minded group of individuals through which such reflective work can be fostered, challenged, and supported. It is suggested that in Western society, we are trained to consider conversations about race, class, or sexuality as "impolite" topics and as such often do not have the language for discussion (American Psychological Association 2003). Without doing individual work, providers run the risk of appearing uncomfortable or dismissive of a patient's experience, which is unlikely to improve the patient's sense that he or she has been able to fully disclose the experience in a way that makes him or her feel heard and understood.

People from minority communities do describe a desire to share their experiences of discrimination and to have the account be heard and believed. To talk about an experience of discrimination and then be made to feel as though this experience is uniquely theirs alone, subjective in nature, and unlikely to have truly happened (Pollack et al. 2012) is detrimental and furthers distrust of the health care system. This kind of experience may result from conversations with individuals who are uncomfortable with the topic at hand and so unintentionally minimize the patient's experience in order to decrease their own discomfort (American Psychological Association 2003) or from conversations with people who do not belong to the same community as the patient and generally have had positive and nondiscriminatory experiences in similar situations. These types of conversation may, in fact, deter the patient from returning to receive care or may further worsen feelings of isolation, anger, distrust, or low mood by virtue of the patient's feeling unheard or feeling as though his or her experience is "all in [my] head."

Having conversations about patient experiences of discrimination is challenging and can bring up many difficult feelings in a provider. Such feelings can be addressed by using models that support individual self-reflection, by inviting speakers to provide anti-oppression training to teams, or by developing a group of individuals who are able to support one another (Beder et al. 2015; Lam et al. 2016; Nyblade et al. 2009). Unfortunately, we know that many of our patients are suffering, often in silence, from repeated experiences of both subtle and overt discrimination. Although making efforts to address these difficulties can feel like uncharted waters for providers and health care organizations, such efforts, when done in a way that is supportive and demonstrates positive regard for the patient experience, is the most ethical way to address the systemic discrimination so many face.

In some ways, these conversations may occur more easily with older adults. Some unimpaired elderly individuals appear to be more resilient to traumas than are younger persons (Sakauye and Nininger, in press). This has been called the *wisdom of age* (Meeks and Jeste 2009). Additionally, as a group, older minorities are less likely to respond with anger and rage at injustices. They often respond with a calm acceptance of racism as a realization that prejudicial issues are unfair but do not define one's identity and cannot be corrected through anger and lashing out (Sakauye 2004, 2011). The older patient may, however, be more critical of professionals who they feel are not open or understanding (Gitlin et al. 2012).

Training in cultural sensitivity and competency should start with information about the minority group with whom the therapist is working and an awareness of the common stereotypes associated with the group (Hays 1996). The therapist's supervisor should be on the lookout for internal inconsistencies that can provide evidence of bias, such as nonverbal cues of distance, difficulty establishing a treatment alliance, an inner sense of irritability or boredom on the part of the therapist, dislike for the patient, a feeling on the part of the patient that the therapist does not understand him or her, lack of practitioner recall regarding details about the patient, incongruities between the therapist's view of the patient and what is in the literature, or a differing opinion from colleagues. Individual supervision for the provider may be helpful for obtaining an objective perspective.

Newer frameworks of cultural competence ask practitioners not only to be aware of individual-level factors affecting culture and health but also to attend to the larger environmental, social, and political factors at play (Betancourt et al. 2002; Kirmayer et al. 2011; Nyblade et al. 2009). Such a framework is often given the name *cultural safety*, wherein providing culturally competent care extends beyond the interaction between a provider and a patient into the sociopolitical domain.

KEY POINTS

- The population of the United States is rapidly aging and becoming more culturally diverse.
- In light of this increasing diversity, cultural competence is an essential component in providing high-quality health care and minimizing health care disparities.
- Health care disparities impact not only patient outcomes but also the cost and economics of health care.
- The implementation of cultural competence ultimately aims to improve efficiency, quality, and equity of health care delivery.

QUESTIONS FOR FURTHER THOUGHT

1. True or False: Persons from ethnic minority groups are more likely than whites to interact with the health care system because minority elderly are more likely to have chronic illnesses.

2. True or False: For health care organizations, overall performance improvement is one of the benefits of providing culturally competent health care.

3. True or False: Regarding individual-level competence, ignoring implicit biases can improve hospital performance metrics.

4. True or False: In the context of health care provision, only direct communication needs to be addressed.

5. True or False: A recent American Heart Association study found that cardiovascular disease awareness among American women was significantly lower among Hispanics than whites.

6. Which of the following is *not* one of the main constructs in the Culturally Competent Model of Care?

    A. Cultural awareness.
    B. Cultural knowledge.
    C. Cultural stigma.
    D. Cultural encounters.
    E. Cultural desire.

SUGGESTED READINGS AND WEBSITES

Health Resources and Services Administration: Medically Underserved Areas and Populations (MUA/P). Available at: bhw.hrsa.gov/shortage-designation/muap

PACE (Programs of All-Inclusive Care for the Elderly): Available at: www.medicare.gov/your-medicare-costs/help-paying-costs/pace/pace.html

Substance Abuse and Mental Health Services Administration: Applying the Strategic Prevention Framework: Cultural Competence. Available at: www.samhsa.gov/capt/applying-strategic-prevention/cultural-competence

REFERENCES

American Counseling Association: Cross-cultural competencies and objectives. Alexandria, VA, American Counseling Association, 1992. Available at: www.counseling.org/Resources/Competencies/Cross-Cultural_Competencies_and_Objectives.pdf. Accessed November 24, 2017.

American Psychiatric Association: Diagnostic and Statistical Manual of Mental Disorders, 4th Edition. Washington, DC, American Psychiatric Association, 1994

American Psychiatric Association: Diagnostic and Statistical Manual of Mental Disorders, 5th Edition. Arlington, VA, American Psychiatric Association, 2013

American Psychological Association: Guidelines on multicultural education, training, research, practice and organizational change for psychologists. Am Psychol 58(5):377–402, 2003 12971086

Anderson LM, Scrimshaw SC, Fullilove MT, et al; Task Force on Community Preventive Services: Culturally competent healthcare systems: a systematic review. Am J Prev Med 24(3)(suppl):68–79, 2003 12668199

Beach MC, Price EG, Gary TL, et al: Cultural competence: a systematic review of health care provider educational interventions. Med Care 43(4):356–373, 2005 15778639

Beder M, Batke A, Hamer D, et al: The Transcultural Psychiatry Reading Group: a learner-led approach to cultural psychiatry. Acad Psychiatry 39(6):703–705, 2015 26122353

Betancourt JR, Green AR, Carrillo JE: Cultural Competence in Health Care: Emerging Frameworks and Practical Approaches. New York, The Commonwealth Fund, October 1, 2002. Available at: www.commonwealth-fund.org/publications/fund-reports/2002/oct/cultural-competence-in-health-care--emerging-frameworks-and-practical-approaches. Accessed November 24, 2017.

Betancourt JR, Green AR, Carrillo JE, et al: Defining cultural competence: a practical framework for addressing racial/ethnic disparities in health and health care. Public Health Rep 118(4):293–302, 2003 12815076

Bhui K, Warfa N, Edonya P, et al: Cultural competence in mental health care: a review of model evaluations. BMC Health Serv Res 7(1):15, 2007 17266765

Brach C, Fraser I: Can cultural competency reduce racial and ethnic health disparities? A review and conceptual model. Med Care Res Rev 57(suppl 1):181–217, 2000 11092163

Brach C, Fraser I: Reducing disparities through culturally competent health care: an analysis of the business case. Qual Manag Health Care 10(4):15–28, 2002 12938253

Butler M, McCreedy E, Schwer N et al: Improving Cultural Competence to Reduce Health Disparities (Comparative Effectiveness Reviews, No 170). Rockville, MD, Agency for Healthcare Research and Quality, 2016

Campinha-Bacote J: The process of cultural competence in the delivery of health care services: a model of care. J Transcult Nurs 13(3):181–184, discussion 200–201, 2002 12113146

Christian AH, Rosamond W, White AR, et al: Nine-year trends and racial and ethnic disparities in women's awareness of heart disease and stroke: an American Heart Association national study. J Womens Health (Larchmt) 16(1):68–81, 2007 17274739

Cross T, Bazron B, Dennis K, et al: Towards a Culturally Competent System of Care, Vol 1. Washington, DC, CASSP Technical Assistance Center, Center for Child and Human Development, Georgetown University, 1989

Díaz RM, Ayala G, Bein E, et al: The impact of homophobia, poverty, and racism on the mental health of gay and bisexual Latino men: findings from 3 US cities. Am J Public Health 91(6):927–932, 2001 11392936

Dries DL, Exner DV, Gersh BJ, et al: Racial differences in the outcome of left ventricular dysfunction. N Engl J Med 340(8):609–616, 1999 10029645

Georgetown University Health Policy Institute: Cultural competence in health care: is it important for people with chronic conditions? (Issue Brief No 5), Washington, DC, Georgetown University, 2004. Available at: https://hpi.georgetown.edu/agingsociety/pubhtml/cultural/cultural.html. Accessed November 24, 2017.

Gitlin LN, Chernett NL, Dennis MP, et al: Identification of and beliefs about depressive symptoms and preferred treatment approaches among community-living older African Americans. Am J Geriatr Psychiatry 20(11):973–984, 2012 22643600

Hall M-B, Carter-Francique AR, Lloyd S, et al: Bias within: examining the role of cultural competence perceptions in mammography adherence. SAGE Open 5(1), 2015

Hays PA: Addressing the complexities of culture and gender in counseling. J Couns Dev 74:332–338, 1996

Institute of Medicine: Unequal Treatment: Confronting Racial and Ethnic Disparities in Health Care. Washington, DC, National Academies Press, 2003

Johnson RL, Saha S, Arbelaez JJ, et al: Racial and ethnic differences in patient perceptions of bias and cultural competence in health care. J Gen Intern Med 19(2):101–110, 2004 15009789

The Joint Commission: Advancing Effective Communication, Cultural Competence, and Patient- and Family-Centered Care: A Roadmap for Hospitals. Oakbrook Terrace, IL, The Joint Commission, 2010. Available at: www.jointcommission.org/assets/1/6/ARoadmapforHospitalsfinal version727.pdf. Accessed November 25, 2017.

Kendler KS: Toward a scientific psychiatry nosology: strengths and limitations. Arch Gen Psychiatry 47(10):969–973, 1990 2222134

Kirmayer LJ: Rethinking cultural competence. Transcult Psychiatry 49(2):149–164, 2012 22508634

Kirmayer LJ, Narasiah L, Munoz M, et al; Canadian Collaboration for Immigrant and Refugee Health (CCIRH): Common mental health problems in immigrants and refugees: general approach in primary care. CMAJ 183(12):E959–E967, 2011 20603342

Lam JS, Gajaria A, Matthews DM, et al: Bridging cultural psychiatry and global mental health: a resident-led initiative. Acad Psychiatry 40(4):729–730, 2016 27217035

Lehman D, Fenza P, Hollinger-Smith L: Diversity and Cultural Competency in Health Care Settings: A Mather LifeWays Orange Paper. 2012. Available at: www.scribd.com/document/279603243/Diversity-and-Cultural-Competency-in-Health-Care-Settings. Accessed November 25, 2017.

McLaughlin KA, Hatzenbuehler ML, Keyes KM: Responses to discrimination and psychiatric disorders among black, Hispanic, female, and lesbian, gay, and bisexual individuals. Am J Public Health 100(8):1477–1484, 2010 20558791

Meeks TW, Jeste DV: Neurobiology of wisdom: a literature overview. Arch Gen Psychiatry 66(4):355–365, 2009 19349305

Meyers KSH: Racial and Ethnic Health Disparities: Influences, Actors, and Policy Opportunities. Oakland, CA, Kaiser Permanente Institute for Health Policy, 2007. Available at: www.kpihp.org/wp-content/uploads/2012/12/Meyers-IHP_Disparities-Influences-Actors-031907.pdf. Accessed May 11, 2018.

National Association of Social Workers: Standards and Indicators for Cultural Competence in Social Work Practice. Washington, DC, National Association of Social Workers, 2015. Available at: www.socialworkers.org/Link Click.aspx?fileticket=7dVckZAYUmk%3d&portalid=0. Accessed May 11, 2018.

National Quality Forum: A Comprehensive Framework and Preferred Practices for Measuring and Reporting Cultural Competency: A Consensus Report. Washington, DC, National Quality Forum, April 2009. Available at: www.qualityforum.org/Publications/2009/04/A_Comprehensive_Framework_and_Preferred_Practices_for_Measuring_and_Reporting_Cultural_Competency.aspx. Accessed November 25, 2017.

Nyblade L, Stangl A, Weiss E, et al: Combating HIV stigma in health care settings: what works? J Int AIDS Soc 12(1):15, 2009 19660113

Ortman JM, Velkoff VA, Hogan H: An Aging Nation: The Older Population in the United States: Population Estimates and Projections (Current Population Reports, P25-1140). Suitland, MD, U.S. Census Bureau, May 2014. Available at: www.census.gov/prod/2014pubs/p25-1140.pdf. Accessed November 27, 2017.

Pascoe EA, Smart Richman L: Perceived discrimination and health: a meta-analytic review. Psychol Bull 135(4):531–554, 2009 19586161

Pollack G, Newbold BK, Lafreniere G, et al: Discrimination in the doctor's office: immigrant and refugee experiences. Critical Social Work 13(2):60–79, 2012

Quach T, Nuru-Jeter A, Morris P, et al: Experiences and perceptions of medical discrimination among a multiethnic sample of breast cancer patients in the greater San Francisco Bay Area, California. Am J Public Health 102(5):1027–1034, 2012 22420791

Renzaho AM, Romios P, Crock C, et al: The effectiveness of cultural competence programs in ethnic minority patient-centered health care—a systematic review of the literature. Int J Qual Health Care 25(3):261–269, 2013 23343990

Sakauye KM: Ethnocultural aspects of aging in mental health, in Comprehensive Textbook of Geriatric Psychiatry, 3rd Edition. Edited by Sadavoy J, Sarvik LF, Grossberg GT, et al. New York, WW Norton, 2004, pp 225–250

Sakauye KM: Cultural issues, in Principles and Practice of Geriatric Psychiatry, 2nd Edition. Edited by Agronin ME, Maletta GJ. Philadelphia, PA, Wolters Kluwer, 2011, pp 225–250

Sakauye KM, Nininger J: Trauma in late life, in Trauma and Stressor-Related Disorders. Edited by Stoddard F, Benedek D, Milad M, et al. New York, Oxford University Press (in press)

Seltzer JA, Yahirun JJ: Diversity in Older Age: The Elderly in Changing Economic and Family Contexts. Providence, RI, U.S. 2010 Project, Brown University, November 6, 2013. Available at: https://s4.ad.brown.edu/Projects/Diversity/Data/Report/report11062013.pdf. Accessed November 25, 2017.

Sharma A, Colvin-Adams M, Yancy CW: Heart failure in African Americans: disparities can be overcome. Cleve Clin J Med 81(5):301–311, 2014 24789589

Smedley BD, Stith AY, Nelson AR: Unequal Treatment: Confronting Racial and Ethnic Disparities in Health Care. Washington, DC, National Academies Press, 2003

Truong M, Paradies Y, Priest N: Interventions to improve cultural competency in healthcare: a systematic review of reviews. BMC Health Serv Res 14:99, 2014 24589335

Tucker CM, Herman KC, Pedersen TR, et al: Cultural sensitivity in physician-patient relationships: perspectives of an ethnically diverse sample of low-income primary care patients. Med Care 41(7):859–870, 2003 12835610

U.S. Census Bureau: Annual Estimates of the Resident Population by Sex, Single Year of Age, Race Alone or in Combination, and Hispanic Origin for the United States: April 1, 2010 to July 1, 2014. Suitland, MD, U.S. Census Bureau, June 2015. Available at: https://factfinder.census.gov/faces/tableservices/jsf/pages/productview.xhtml?pid=PEP_2016_PEPALL5N&prodType=table. Accessed May 11, 2018.

U.S. Department of Health and Human Services: National Standards for Culturally and Linguistically Appropriate Services in Health Care: Final Report. Rockville, MD, Office of Minority Health, 2001. Available at: http://minorityhealth.hhs.gov/assets/pdf/checked/finalreport.pdf. Accessed November 27, 2017.

U.S. Department of Health and Human Services: 2016 National Healthcare Quality and Disparities Report. Rockville, MD, Agency for Healthcare Research and Quality, May 2016. Available at: www.ahrq.gov/research/findings/nhqrdr/nhqdr16/index.html. Accessed May 17, 2018.

Villablanca AC, Slee C, Lianov L, et al: Outcomes of a clinic-based educational intervention for cardiovascular disease prevention by race, ethnicity, and urban/rural status. J Womens Health (Larchmt) 25(11):1174–1186, 2016 27356155

Vincent GK, Velkoff VA: The Next Four Decades: The Older Population in the United States: 2010 to 2050 (Current Population Reports, P25-1138). Suitland, MD, U.S. Census Bureau, May 2010. Available at: www.census.gov/prod/2010pubs/p25-1138.pdf. Accessed November 27, 2017.

Weech-Maldonado R, Dreachslin JL, Brown J, et al: Cultural competency assessment tool for hospitals: evaluating hospitals' adherence to the Culturally and Linguistically Appropriate Services standards. Health Care Manage Rev 37(1):54–66, 2012a 21934511

Weech-Maldonado R, Elliott M, Pradhan R, et al: Can hospital cultural competency reduce disparities in patient experiences with care? Med Care 50(suppl):S48–S55, 2012b 23064277

Weech-Maldonado R, Dreachslin JL, Epané JP, et al: Hospital cultural competency as a systematic organizational intervention: key findings from the National Center for Healthcare Leadership Diversity Demonstration project. Health Care Manage Rev October 25, 2016 [Epub ahead of print] 27782970

Wierenga KL, Dekker RL, Lennie TA, et al: African American race is associated with poorer outcomes in heart failure patients. West J Nurs Res (July):1–15, 2016 27470676

CHAPTER 2

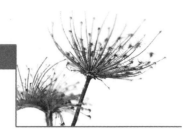

Cultural Competence in Geriatric Psychiatry

TEACHING AND EVALUATIVE METHODS

Ken Sakauye, M.D.

Shuo Sally He, M.D., M.P.H.

Ebony Dix, M.D.

Raissa Tanqueco, M.D.

Iqbal Ahmed, M.D., FRCPsych

Learning Objectives

Be able to apply the following Accreditation Council for Graduate Medical Education (ACGME) core competencies to cultural psychiatry and, more particularly, to the ethnic older adult group with whom one is working:

1. Patient care

2. Medical knowledge

3. Practice-based learning and improvement

4. Interpersonal and communication skills

5. Professionalism

6. Systems-based practice

The concept of cultural competency plays an important role in providing quality care and positive outcomes, gathering subjective data about a patient that may ultimately impact outcomes. When initially interviewing a patient, it is standard for a clinician to obtain a psychosocial, cultural/ethnic, and family history. This enables the clinician to identify major psychosocial factors impacting a patient's medical health and develop a cultural formulation and accurate differential diagnosis. Also relevant to patient care is how the clinician's awareness and understanding of the patient's psychosocial and ethnic background, as well as awareness of how the clinician's own background, may impact his or her attitudes toward a patient.

One can think of each Accreditation Council for Graduate Medical Education (ACGME) core competency (Table 2–1) as a component skill required by trainees because they all provide *patient care*.

TABLE 2–1.   ACGME core competencies

1. Patient care

2. Medical knowledge

3. Practice-based learning and improvement

4. Interpersonal and communication skills

5. Professionalism

6. Systems-based practice

Note.   ACGME = Accreditation Council for Graduate Medical Education.

Medical knowledge is a competency that includes a clinician's ability to have an adequate fund of knowledge about cultural, ethnic, and socioeconomic factors that are relevant to a patient's psychopathology. Clinicians apply this knowledge and clinical principles to patient care.

Practice-based learning and improvement require trainees to improve on patient care through continued review of the medical literature, self-evaluation, educating others, and implementing quality improvement. This may include improving one's knowledge base about particular evidence in the literature regarding the treatment modalities of certain conditions within specific cultural/ethnic frameworks. Clinicians improve their understanding and knowledge of certain cultural beliefs or practices that may impact treatment. It is then important for clinicians to educate other clinicians and apply their knowledge to implementation of quality improvement measures to provide more culturally competent care.

Interpersonal and communication skills are a critical area of patient care, especially in a patient population that is ethnically, culturally, and socioeconomically diverse. Communicating effectively with a patient requires that a clinician be able to incorporate his or her awareness and knowledge of psychosocial and cultural attributes that are unique to a patient. The clinician should demonstrate caring, respectful behaviors that supersede self-interest when interacting with patients and peers in the workplace. This ties into professionalism as well.

Professionalism embodies the qualities of compassion, integrity, and responsiveness to patient needs. It includes a commitment to punctuality, confidentiality, patient rights, and the ethical principles that apply to provision of excellent care.

Systems-based practice requires the clinician to understand the factors that affect cross-cultural interactions in geriatric mental health care. This includes the cultural backgrounds of providers and patients and the culture of the community or setting. Through application of this competency, clinicians learn to appreciate the organization of mental health systems that serve specific ethnic or sociocultural groups and plan individual patient care accordingly. This ultimately assists patients in dealing with system complexities.

A work group tasked by the Association of American Medical Colleges (AAMC) attempted to narrow the scope of geriatric competencies into fewer core competencies by subdividing tasks into eight domains: medication management; self-care capacity; falls, balance and gait disorders; hospital care for elders; cognitive and behavioral disorders; atypical presentation of disease; health care planning and promotion; and palliative care (Leipzig et al. 2009). These competency domains were identified to provide graduating medical students with specific areas of competency that are essential in the daily practice of working with geriatric patients. These defined competencies are what residency program directors expect incoming interns to have successfully completed during medical school training.

The work group created three additional domains that are central to cultural competency (Table 2–2). Within each domain, observable behaviors were identified that demonstrate cultural competency in older adult patients. These are also relevant to the ACCME core competencies listed in Table 2–1.

There are many curriculum guides, textbooks, and recommended readings on cultural competence, but few are specific to geriatric minority populations. Available free online curricula that are specific to geriatric psychiatry include Stanford University's Ethnogeriatrics curriculum (https://geriatrics.stanford.edu); the American Psychiatric Association

TABLE 2–2. Minimum competencies for additional geriatric psychiatry cultural domains

Domain	Behaviors demonstrating competency
Awareness of the individual's cultural background and cultural values	Applies the Cultural Formulation Interview and Geriatric Supplement (American Psychiatric Association 2013) to a minority older patient Demonstrates knowledge of the patient's culture and recognizes the relevance of the patient's experiences
Establishment of a treatment alliance	Communicates effectively and is respectful of behaviors that supersede self-interest Invites mutual respect
Appropriate modifications to psychotherapy and/or family work	Can conceptualize and describe approach

(APA) Ethnic Minority Elderly Curriculum, available from the American Association for Geriatric Psychiatry (AAGP; www.aagponline.org/clientuploads/08cultcompcur.pdf); and the California Endowment Cultural Competence Education for Health Care Professionals (www.vdh.virginia.gov/ohpp/clasact/documents/clasact/general/managerguide.pdf).

CULTURAL COMPETENCE WITH MULTIPLE MINORITY GROUPS

Is it possible for a clinician to be culturally competent with all minority groups? The short answer is no. There are well over 100 ethnic groups in the United States, with wide diversity within each ethnic group. Although many geriatric patients from different ethnic groups are U.S.-born, some are non-English speaking. Some are assimilated; others are not. Clinicians must strive to be culturally competent with groups that might be seen regularly in one's practice.

A starting point to a general understanding of cultural backgrounds is the ambitious *Harvard Encyclopedia of American Ethnic Groups* (Thernstrom 1980), which provides the background of major ethnic groups in the United States up to 1980. This encyclopedia covers more than 100 ethnic groups, dealing with common geographic origins, race, language or dialect, migration, arrival, settlement and employment patterns, shared traditions, values and symbols, literature and folklore, music, food preferences, special interests with regard to politics, institutions that specifically serve and maintain the group, kinship, behavior, culture, religion, education, intergroup relations, internal sense of distinctiveness, and external perception of distinctiveness. Additional groups that have arrived in the United States as the result of more recent worldwide conflicts and disasters are not covered in this text. These newer immigrant groups will require similar analysis for cultural competence.

TEACHING METHODS

Several different teaching methods can be used not only to provide knowledge in the area of various cultural backgrounds but also to increase cultural sensitivity, ultimately leading to cultural competency. Some of the teaching methods suggested are didactic, whereas others are experiential techniques, such as use of bibliographic and video resources, small-group learning, clinical teaching, and research-based teaching. Most of these techniques have been well described and used in the comprehensive ethnogeriatrics curriculum developed by Stanford (Yeo 2010).

Didactic Methods

Didactic approaches to basic cross-cultural psychiatry should include the following concepts: culture; ethnicity; genetic issues; race; diversity; disadvantaged populations; immigration issues; acculturation; cultural sensitivity; cultural competency; cultural formulation; diagnostic issues; diagnostic bias; use of interpreters; treatment issues, including ethnopsychopharmacology; principles of psychotherapy; systems issues such as attitudes toward health, health care, and health care givers, accessibility of care, and health care utilization; and culturally competent systems. Most of these concepts are described in texts on cross-cultural psychiatry, including a number published by American Psychiatric Publishing (Gaw 2001; Lim 2015; Streltzer 2017; Tseng and Streltzer 2001, 2004).

Didactic methods of teaching cross-cultural geriatric psychiatry should include both general concepts and specifics, especially as they relate to the different ethnic groups on such topics as the following:

- Demographics of ethnic groups, especially the ethnic minority elderly
- Concepts of normal and abnormal aging
- Beliefs about death and dying

- Health care beliefs and behaviors
- Interaction of cultural factors with age factors
- Acculturation issues
- Traditional roles of family members
- Concerns of ethnic elders and their families
- Protective factors against and risk factors for mental illness
- Ethnic differences with respect to specific disorders
- Ethnopsychopharmacology and other treatment issues (Chaudhry et al. 2008; Chen et al. 2008)
- Systems issues such as attitudes toward health, health care, and health care givers; accessibility of care; and health care utilization

Most of these issues are covered in Chapters 4–11. General issues related to ethnic elders have also been reviewed by Cohen et al. (2018), Lee and Ahmed (2017), Sakauye (2004), and Takeshita and Ahmed (2004).

Experiential Techniques

Experiential techniques encourage students to examine their own cultural attitudes and values that could affect their interactions with elders from diverse backgrounds. This can be done by assigning the following exercises:

- A paper asking students to examine the influence of their own cultural background on their attitudes toward people of different cultures
- Use of reflection (journaling)
- Reflective narratives about students' own ethnic backgrounds; values; and beliefs about health, health care, the interaction between spirituality and health, and death

Additionally, discussion sessions can be held in which learners are asked to do the following:

- Share the health beliefs of their own families based on cultural and religious backgrounds
- Explore the similarities and differences in their backgrounds
- Respect differing values and beliefs

Videos and Biographical Resources

Elders from diverse ethnic populations can be invited to discuss the important historical events in their lives and health beliefs that they and others of their ethnic group hold. Profiles of elders of various ethnic groups can be viewed in film or video formats. Students then can be asked to place the elders in a specific cohort and discuss the possible influences of the specific culture on their clinical care. Additionally, students can be encouraged to read biographies of ethnic elders. Finally, two generations of elders from the same ethnic population can be compared in terms of the responses to the health care system based on their historical experiences.

For example, Japanese Americans are often viewed as a model of assimilation, but clinicians may see this group in a different light after viewing a 2010 Japanese television series called *99 Years of Love*. This program describes the bittersweet reunion of two siblings, one trapped in Japan during World War II and one who stayed in the United States and was sent to an internment camp as a child. This is a positive model that could be juxtaposed with *Who's Going to Pay for These Donuts, Anyway?*, a 1993 documentary about an elderly Japanese American man with schizophrenia who had his first break at the time of internment. This program shows the effect of a cultural trauma and the disruption it caused to one family. These types of documentaries and docudramas can help clinicians understand the modal experiences of a group with which they are working and helps create empathy. The most information is available about African American elderly and the effect of prejudice and discrimination.

Clinical Teaching

Education in cultural psychiatry must address two areas: 1) patient-specific knowledge (how to understand and deal with the patient more effectively) and 2) dealing with the clinician's own unconscious biases toward other races and/or cultures.

Patient-Specific Knowledge

To prepare residents for clinical exposures, medical students should receive an orientation to patient-specific cultural competence early in their training. The APA and AAGP addressed patient-specific knowledge of culture in their initial "Curriculum Resource Guide for Cultural Competence" (American Psychiatric Association/American Association for Geriatric Psychiatry 1997). Being aware that most psychiatric residents may not have social science backgrounds, the initial recommendation of the APA/AAGP curriculum guide was to focus the orientation course on the following topics (American Psychiatric Association/American Association for Geriatric Psychiatry 1997):

- Introduction to cultural and sociopolitical considerations (overarching themes, including types of data for which controlled studies are not possible)

- Assimilation and cultural issues, worldviews, and healing beliefs
- Racial and cultural identity development and the effects of prejudice
- Culturally fair assessments and test instruments that compensate for low educational attainment, language effects, and differences in communication styles
- Minority family issues (affiliative patterns, marital status, concepts of family obligation, social structures)
- Cultural formulation
- Psychotherapy issues (e.g., the unique aspects of therapy for minority elderly compared with younger cohorts)

Ethnocentrism

Ethnocentrism (ethnocentric bias) is a term used since the late 1880s for the tendency to judge another culture solely by the values and standards of one's own culture. Countertransference, the result of the patient's influence on the physician's unconscious feelings, describes a similar phenomenon. A more recent term is *relational reality*, in which beliefs are based on actual experiences or learning but may not be accurately generalizable. These two terms are more commonly called *prejudice*. No one thinks they are prejudiced, even when others think they are, but inattention or denial of a lack of awareness or unconscious mental processes may cause problems in working with elderly minority populations.

Amadio (2014) reviewed studies of unconscious prejudice. These studies showed activation of frontal and limbic areas related to negative emotions or fear when white subjects were exposed to black faces, with nonactivation of empathy and mentalizing areas of the brain. This reaction was not seen when the same subjects were exposed to white faces. This is probably learned behavior that then becomes internalized into an individual's worldview. Clinicians should try to approach this type of bias logically and address it systematically. Tables 2–3, 2–4, and 2–5 present aspects of bias that should be taught in clinical supervision (Dewald 1969; Jost et al. 2008).

IDEAS FOR TRAINING MODALITIES

Individualized Training

1. Increase awareness of the individual's cultural background and cultural values.

TABLE 2–3.   Signs of bias or prejudice in the clinician

Negative patient responses to the clinician (e.g., nonverbal cues of distancing)

Problems in establishing a treatment alliance

Acting "out of character" or being unable to empathize with the individual

An inner sense of irritability or boredom with the patient

Not liking the patient

Jumping to conclusions

Poor memory about the patient

Incongruities between the clinician's views and what is in the literature

Differing opinion from colleagues (i.e., the clinician's beliefs are idiosyncratic)

TABLE 2–4.   Possible sources of clinician bias

Belief is based on actual experiences in interactions but is not really characteristic of a race or culture (focus of personal projections)

Belief is based only on what the clinician was told or learned, although this information is not accurate

Belief is widely held in the dominant culture and therefore may not be readily questioned

TABLE 2–5.   Techniques for overcoming bias

Learn as much as possible about the culture and experiences of the patient

Broaden one's understanding of racism, ethnocentrism, and perceived oppression and disenfranchisement that affect people of color

Become sensitive to potential developmental effects of prejudice on personality and worldviews

Apply qualitative research methods to the clinical situation

- Discuss the DSM-5 Cultural Formulation Interview (CFI; American Psychiatric Association 2013) and apply it to specific cases. The CFI focuses on the patient's view of the illness, the patient's own attempts at treatment; the people to whom he or she turns for help; and potential barriers to treatment, including unwillingness to work with the interviewer. This is a marked departure from DSM-IV (American Psychiatric Association 1994), which viewed cultural issues as unusual culture-bound syndromes. Use the CFI and its supplementary modules (American Psychiatric Association 2017; Lewis-Fernández et al. 2016) to discuss how the formulation has changed the understanding and management of cases. Role-play taking turns as patient, caregiver, and interviewer.

- Create opportunities for medical students, residents, and fellows to interview a person of interest (e.g., an elderly patient who emigrated from another country) to understand that person's life history instead of giving the patient a clinical diagnosis. These interviews may be documented in writing, in recorded form (e.g., StoryCorps phone app), or in videos for further discussion.

2. Establish a treatment alliance.

- Practice effective communication with mutual respect and a professional manner.

- Practice communicating with and educating geriatric patients and family members regarding their mental health diagnosis, management, and treatment plan in a culturally appropriate manner while eliciting patients' and families' views of illness.

- Discuss how to work appropriately with interpreters.

3. Make appropriate modifications to psychotherapy and/or family work.

- Have students conduct an assessment using an interpreter, followed up with discussion of the benefits, difficulties, and strategies of using an interpreter to promote communication.

- Provide role modeling by faculty in professional interactions with patients, families, colleagues, staff, consultees, students, trainees, and employees.

- Conduct geriatric assessments with culturally diverse older adults and elicit feedback from the elders and their family members.

- Provide clinical supervision to teach cultural sensitivity and observe resident interactions in dealing with patients, families, and other caregivers to ensure that these interactions are done with cultural sensitivity.

Group Training

- Hold cultural psychiatry case conferences with different themes for discussion (e.g., sociopolitical factors such as health care access, treatment of dementia, and psychopharmacological considerations).
- Invite speakers with a cultural competency training background to teach residents and fellows and discuss concerns.
- Obtain resources such as poetry, books, religious texts, and music from an ethnic community for a training program and group discussions.

Continuing Educational Opportunities

- Create training videos pertaining to specific topics of cultural competency in working with the elderly (e.g., how to use interpreters properly) to be disseminated to training program and other team members.
- Create and use a cultural competency training manual or toolkit for training current and/or incoming residents and fellows.
- Create a teaching committee in cultural competency for a training program or modify an existing curriculum such as the Cultural Competence Education from the AAMC (Association of American Medical Colleges 2005)
- Provide "lunch and learn" opportunities for staff. Invite speakers (including patients and caregivers) from diverse communities to talk about their ethnic group and cultural experiences or invite representatives from an organization to talk about their best practices working with a diverse group of people.
- Offer cultural sensitivity training on a regular basis to address issues associated with literacy, language barriers, family support, the need for respect, traditions, and alternative health and illness remedies.
- Exhibit information on cultural competence in order to create a culture of awareness.
- Provide opportunities and reimbursement for staff to attend professional meetings and conferences.
- Create collaborative monthly meetings to discuss providing culturally competent care to geriatric patients. These sessions can be led by residents or fellows, social workers, geriatricians, or other professionals.

Evidence-Based Intervention

- Ask group participants to perform a literature search to find up-to-date, evidence-based intervention trainings in cultural competency pertaining to care of geriatric patients.
- Administer a cultural competency assessment.
- Have group participants analyze census data and report the variations or lack of information within specifically defined populations of the elderly (e.g., by gender, ethnicity, geographic location, or insurance status).
- Evaluate changes in outcomes (e.g., attitude, knowledge, skills, behaviors) after implementation of a cultural competency training curriculum and continue to modify training programs.

Systems-Based Considerations

- Have the resident or fellow identify a personal experience with a patient who is from a cultural background different from his or her own background. Then, identify systems-based barriers or issues related to cultural competency and discuss ways to address or overcome those barriers.
- Analyze indicators of cultural competency within the health care system of the residents' or fellows' own communities.
- Create a cultural competency work group or committee within the training program, hospital, or organization and work to integrate it as a core value of the organization. Assess the organization for barriers to cultural competency and provide recommendations for how to provide culturally competent care.
- Research current resources and guidelines for cultural competency and apply them to the geriatric population (Georgetown University Health Policy Institute 2004; Lehman et al. 2015).
- Learn about current organizational, state, and federal standards and recommendations for cultural competency as well as patients' rights.
- Identify and encourage involvement with the residency or training program, hospital organization, local community organizations or advocacy groups, and/or state and federal agencies to assess for cultural competence and implement policy changes pertaining to the geriatric population of a specific racial/ethnic group or population of interest.
- Discuss public policy and public advocacy issues related to the identified population of interest (e.g., as defined by socioeconomic status, racial/ethnic group, or insurance issues).

- Identify and discuss ways to reduce health disparities in access to psychiatric care for the elderly.

Research-Based Teaching

- Perform a literature search to find up-to-date, evidence-based intervention and modalities of training on cultural competency pertaining to care of geriatric patients.
- Identify gaps in knowledge and perform needs assessment on topics related to cultural competency in geriatric psychiatry that require further research.
- Consider a literature search focusing on types of outcomes impacted by the provision of culturally competent care (e.g., patient outcome measures, access and health care utilization measures) (Truong et al. 2014).
- Conduct a journal club to discuss papers with particular issues pertaining to cultural considerations in geriatric psychiatry.
- Develop and support research projects involving sociocultural considerations, family system beliefs, health beliefs, or other related topics on cultural competency of elderly patient care.
- Consider recruitment of research participants who are elderly and from ethnic minorities.
- Develop consent forms that are culturally relevant.
- Develop culturally relevant research and assessment instruments.
- Consider collaboration with interpreters, local community organizations and their members, or expert advisers when designing and conducting research with a group of interest.
- Seek out and discuss innovative, culturally appropriate solutions in helping with assessment and treatment of geriatric patients.
- Encourage discussion and writeup for publication of cases related to cultural competency in geriatric patients.

Modules on Specific Ethnic Groups

- Interview ethnic elders on the help they give and receive or other specific topics and present the results of the interviews in class to compare and discuss similarities and differences.
- Invite a traditional medicine practitioner or visit a community clinic that works with many patients from a particular sociocultural group to discuss cultural conceptions of illness, treatment, and health.
- Observe a case conference of an interdisciplinary team meeting with a focus on an older ethnic minority patient.

- Encourage participation or observation through grand rounds and/ or conferences to develop and reinforce insights into conceptions of illness and treatment approaches.
- Augment assigned readings, lectures, and discussion with the following activities and resources.
    - Download the latest data on life expectancy and mortality rates for elders from different ethnic populations from websites (e.g., www.agid.acl.gov) and make comparisons.
    - View online cultural competency training modules such as Cultural Competence and Clinical Care (New York State Office of Mental Health 2015) and discuss adaptations needed to apply these modules to geriatric populations.
    - Participate in group projects that address ethnic groups and differences in diseases such as depression, dementia, and suicide; differences in treatment approaches, such as use of psychotropic drugs; and the risks of complications such as tardive dyskinesia, diabetes, hypercholesterolemia, and stroke. Discuss additional concerns that may be unique to the elderly, such as sexual practices, physical illness, end-of-life concerns, or other culturally important values.
    - Visit a local nursing home, personal care home, or day program for an older ethnic group for a prearranged question-and-answer session talking about the history of that group's health and health care.
    - Participate in a field trip to a historical museum dealing with a specific ethnic group to see films, pictorial displays, and other objects pertinent to the health history of the ethnic group.

EVALUATION

The method of evaluation for practitioners is a self-assessment. The approach should be similar to the maintenance of certification approach, which has two components: 1) evidence for continuing medical education (CME) in the area of evaluation, consisting of either CME activities or peer-reviewed publications in the area and 2) proof of competency around a case, documented in a note or and/or discussions with colleagues.

For trainees, ACGME core competencies also apply to each domain, but usually they have been applied in a more general way. For example, excellent patient care may refer to the final outcome and not to a particular skill set in one of the domains. A sample rating form using the ACGME competencies is available in the appendix to this chapter. An observational structured clinical examination, similar to the American Board of Psychiatry and Neurology oral examinations, could also be developed.

Evaluation of student understanding of culturally appropriate health care is best evaluated via essay questions or written reports. Essay questions can be used to evaluate trainees' understanding of the sources and data limitations. This format allows the student to explore more fully differences in what constitutes culturally competent care. In addition, evaluations can take the form of objective tests for retention of information or assigned papers that reflect increased self-knowledge of one's own cultural attitudes and values. The assigned papers could be in the form of individual or group projects. Use of the Geriatric Psychiatry Cultural Competency Evaluation Form (see appendix to this chapter) can document specific areas of competence.

KEY POINTS

- Teaching methods should include didactic methods, experiential techniques, and supervision.
- Signs of bias that one must always be aware of are negative patient responses such as distancing, problems establishing a treatment alliance, the clinician not liking the patient, jumping to conclusions, poor clinician memory about the patient, incongruities between the clinician's views and the literature, and differing opinions from colleagues.
- Bias is not always the same as prejudice. We all have unconscious biases and must be aware when they become a barrier to understanding and empathy.
- Specific didactic methods for teaching cultural competency include use of ethnic-specific modules and videos. Specific evidence-based training interventions include literature searches, analysis of census data, and evaluations of changes in outcomes after cultural competency training. Competency can be evaluated using the Geriatric Psychiatry Cultural Competency Evaluation Form.

QUESTIONS FOR FURTHER THOUGHT

1. Name four essential practice-based learning and improvement techniques for cultural competence.

2. An elderly African American Vietnam era veteran has trauma-related symptoms of hypervigilance, anxiety, and nightmares that worsened in late life. A white psychiatry resident who is usually sympathetic with patients minimizes the effect of reported race baiting and threats by saying that the patient is just trying to get free benefits. In what ways does this vignette demonstrate unconscious biases that are affecting care?

3. How might one learn about another culture without working directly with that group?

4. A work group tasked by the Association of Medical Colleges (AAMC) recommends how many curricular domains for cultural competency for medical students?

    A. Three.
    B. Five.
    C. Eight.
    D. Twelve.

5. True or False: There is increased activation of the mentalizing areas of the brain during exposure of black faces to white subjects.

SUGGESTED READINGS AND WEBSITES

American Psychiatric Association/American Association for Geriatric Psychiatry: Curriculum Resource Guide for Cultural Competence: A Joint Project. Washington, DC, American Psychiatric Association and American Association for Geriatric Psychiatry, 1997

Gilbert MJ (ed): A Manager's Guide to Cultural Competence Education for Health Care Professionals. Woodland Hills, CA, California Endowment, 2003. Available at: www.vdh.virginia.gov/ohpp/clasact/documents/clasact/general/managerguide.pdf.

Yeo G: Ethnogeriatrics overview: introduction. Stanford, CA, Stanford School of Medicine, Stanford University, 2010. Available at: https://geriatrics.stanford.edu/culturemed/overview/introduction.html.

References

Amadio D: The neuroscience of prejudice and stereotyping. Nat Rev Neurosci 15(10):670–682, 2014 25186236

American Psychiatric Association: Diagnostic and Statistical Manual of Mental Disorders, 4th Edition. Washington, DC, American Psychiatric Association, 1994

American Psychiatric Association: Cultural formulation, in Diagnostic and Statistical Manual of Mental Disorders, 5th Edition. Arlington, VA, American Psychiatric Association, 2013, pp 749–759

American Psychiatric Association: Supplementary modules to the core Cultural Formulation Interview. Educational Resources: Online Assessment Measures. Arlington, VA, American Psychiatric Association, 2017. Available at: www.psychiatry.org/psychiatrists/practice/dsm/educational-resources/assessment-measures. Accessed December 5, 2017.

American Psychiatric Association/American Association for Geriatric Psychiatry: Curriculum Resource Guide for Cultural Competence: A Joint Project. Washington, DC, American Psychiatric Association and American Association for Geriatric Psychiatry, 1997

Association of American Medical Colleges: Cultural Competence Education. Washington, DC, Association of American Medical Colleges, 2005. Available at: www.aamc.org/download/54338/data. Accessed December 4, 2017.

Chaudhry I, Neelam K, Duddu V, et al: Ethnicity and psychopharmacology. J Psychopharmacol 22(6):673–680, 2008 18308818

Chen CH, Chen CY, Lin KM: Ethnopsychopharmacology. Int Rev Psychiatry 20(5):452–459, 2008 19012131

Cohen C, Elmouchtar M, Ahmed I: Working with elderly persons across cultures, in Textbook of Cultural Psychiatry, 2nd Edition. Edited by Bhugra D, Bhui K. New York, Cambridge University Press, 2018, pp 552–569

Dewald PA: Counter-transference, in Psychotherapy: A Dynamic Approach, 2nd Edition. New York, Basic Books, 1969, pp 254–262

Gaw AC (ed): Concise Guide to Cross-Cultural Psychiatry. Washington, DC, American Psychiatric Press, 2001

Georgetown University Health Policy Institute: Cultural Competence in Health Care: Is It Important for People With Chronic Conditions? Washington, DC, Health Policy Institute, Georgetown University, February 2004. Available at: https://hpi.georgetown.edu/agingsociety/pubhtml/cultural/cultural.html. Accessed December 6, 2017.

Jost JT, Ledgerwood A, Hardin CD: Shared reality, system justification, and the relational basis of ideological beliefs. Soc Personal Psychol Compass 2(1):171–186, 2008

Lee J, Ahmed I: Geriatric psychopathology, in Culture and Psychopathology: A Guide to Clinical Assessment, 2nd Edition. Edited by Streltzer J. New York, Routledge, 2017, pp 161–168

Lehman D, Fenza P, Hollinger-Smith L: Diversity and Cultural Competency in Health Care Settings. Evanston, IL, Mather LifeWays, September 9, 2015. Available at: www.scribd.com/document/279603243/Diversity-and-Cultural-Competency-in-Health-Care-Settings. Accessed December 6, 2017.

Leipzig RM, Granville L, Simpson D, et al: Keeping granny safe on July 1: a consensus on minimum geriatrics competencies for graduating medical students. Acad Med 84(5):604–610, 2009 19704193

Lewis-Fernández R, Aggarwal NK, Hinton L, et al (eds): DSM-5 Handbook on the Cultural Formulation Interview. Arlington, VA, American Psychiatric Association Publishing, 2016

Lim R (ed): Clinical Manual of Cultural Psychiatry, 2nd Edition. Arlington, VA, American Psychiatric Publishing, 2015

New York State Office of Mental Health: Cultural Competence and Clinical Care. Albany, NY, Office of Mental Health, 2015. Available at: www.omh.ny.gov/ omhweb/cultural_competence/clinical_care.html. Accessed December 6, 2017.

Sakauye KM: Ethnocultural aspects of aging in mental health, in Comprehensive Textbook of Geriatric Psychiatry, 3rd Edition. Edited by Sadavoy J, Jarvik LF, Grossberg GT, et al. New York, WW Norton, 2004, pp 225–250

Streltzer J (ed): Culture and Psychopathology: A Guide to Clinical Assessment, 2nd Edition. New York, Routledge, 2017

Takeshita J, Ahmed I: Cultural aspects of geriatric psychiatry, in Culture Competence in Clinical Psychiatry. Edited by Tseng W-S, Streltzer J. Washington, DC, American Psychiatric Publishing, 2004, pp 147–161

Thernstrom S: Harvard Encyclopedia of American Ethnic Groups. Cambridge, MA, Belknap, 1980

Truong M, Paradies Y, Priest N: Interventions to improve cultural competency in healthcare: a systematic review of reviews. BMC Health Serv Res 14:99, 2014 24589335

Tseng W-S, Streltzer J (eds): Culture and Psychotherapy: A Guide to Clinical Practice. Washington, DC, American Psychiatric Press, 2001

Tseng W-S, Streltzer J (eds): Culture Competence in Clinical Psychiatry. Washington, DC, American Psychiatric Publishing, 2004

Yeo G: Ethnogeriatrics overview: introduction. Stanford, CA, Stanford Medicine, Stanford University, 2010. Available at: https://geriatrics.stanford.edu/ culturemed/overview/introduction.html. Accessed December 6, 2017.

Appendix

Geriatric Psychiatry Cultural Competency Evaluation Form

Resident Name:

Attending Evaluator's Name:

Date of Evaluation:

Be as specific as possible, including reports of critical incidents and/or outstanding performance. NA = not applicable, insufficient contact to judge

Unsatisfactory=1   Marginal=2   Satisfactory=3   Excellent=4   Exemplary=5

Patient Care/Clinical Skills

1	2	3	4	5	NA
Interview Skills					
Is incomplete, disorganized, awkward. Lacks focus. Does not take a sociocultural history. Misses important cultural cues from patient.	Obtains basic sociocultural data but often misses significant cultural/ethnic historical findings.	Conducts complete interviews. Solicits data for all elements of sociocultural and ethnic history. May lack logical, flowing sequence or transitions. Some backtracking.	Conducts well-paced, logically sequenced interviews. Rarely misses important findings. Skillfully solicits sensitive data. Shows flexibility in style.	Conducts artful, efficient, focused interviews. Accurately detects subtle or sensitive findings. Handles difficult issues effectively.	

Patient Care/Clinical Skills (continued)

1	2	3	4	5	NA
Diagnosis and Formulation					
Misses major sociocultural problems. Cannot interpret basic data. Unable to correctly identify a working diagnosis without assistance.	Usually identifies the major sociocultural problems correctly. May not integrate all aspects of data. May report data without analysis. Sociocultural problem list is incomplete.	Independently identifies major sociocultural problems. Constructs an accurate multiaxial diagnosis and rudimentary cultural formulation.	Regularly identifies predisposing, precipitating, and maintaining factors, including sociocultural factors. Cultural formulation shows appreciation of interaction between patient's problems and various elements of the formulation. Correctly prioritizes sociocultural problems.	Makes sophisticated biopsychosocial and cultural assessments. Formulation is supported by theoretical framework and/or evidence-based sources of understanding.	

Patient Care/Clinical Skills *(continued)*

1	2	3	4	5	NA
Patient Management					
Unsafe, erroneous, or neglectful practices. May fail to monitor or follow up patients closely. May cause patient distress through cultural insensitivity. Does not apply principles of cultural psychiatry to psychosocial and psychopharmacological treatments.	May have narrow focus in patient care. Does not seem to appreciate sociocultural context of patient care.	Shows sound judgment about sociocultural factors. Incorporates awareness in treatment planning with assistance.	Provides comprehensive care, incorporating ethnic and sociocultural factors. Able to anticipate problems. Effectively handles patient's biopsychological and sociocultural problems independently.	Reasons well in complex or ambiguous sociocultural issues. Shows high level of initiative and independence in monitoring and planning care. Applies preventive interventions before problems arise.	

Specific comments recognizing excellent performance or areas for improvement in patient care/clinical skills:

Knowledge

1	2	3	4	5	NA
Major deficiencies in basic concepts and key sociocultural facts. Minimal interest in learning. Does not understand complex relationships and mechanisms of disease and treatment, including effects of culture and ethnicity on psychosocial and psychopharmacological treatment.	Weak knowledge base. Many gaps in fundamental facts.	Consistently demonstrates an adequate fund of knowledge. Applies basic science and clinical principles to patient care.	Strong fund of knowledge. Considerable, expanded understanding of psychopathology and sociocultural factors in normal development, psychopathology, and treatment, both psychosocial and psychopharmacological.	Comprehensive and up-to-date knowledge. Demonstrates strong analytical thinking. Articulates current issues in controversial or unresolved areas of cultural psychiatry, sociology, and anthropology. Supports statements with literature references.	

Specific comments recognizing excellent performance or areas for improvement in knowledge:

Interpersonal and Communication Skills

1	2	3	4	5	NA
With Patients					
Shows insensitivity to patient concerns. Unable to establish rapport. Lacks awareness of cultural factors in communication. Lacks respect for patients' cultural beliefs and values. Not empathic.	Lacks skill in listening and communicating effectively. Difficulty managing boundaries. Has episodes of miscommunication with patients and families due to cultural insensitivity.	Creates and sustains a therapeutic and ethically sound relationship with patients and their families. Communicates effectively, incorporating awareness of sociocultural factors. Demonstrates caring, respectful behaviors that supersede self-interest.	Able to establish a relationship with patients with more difficult sociocultural issues. Demonstrates consistent empathy. Has expanded listening and verbal skills. Overcomes cultural barriers and mistrust.	Creates and sustains therapeutic relationship with patients with very challenging or difficult sociocultural issues. Effectively manages a volatile family meeting. Handles complex boundary issues skillfully. Manages own anxiety well. Shows maturity in use of self.	

Interpersonal and Communication Skills *(continued)*

1	2	3	4	5	NA
With Colleagues					
Insensitive to cultural differences and differences in communication styles. May be the source of complaints by personnel.	Shows difficulty working with others. May show inflexibility, minimal consideration, or lack of respect to cultural differences.	Works effectively with colleagues of all sociocultural backgrounds. Invites mutual respect.	Shows ability to be flexible, compromise, and admit errors. Recognizes the strengths and limits of others' communication styles, beliefs, and values.	Shows high level of teamwork, collegiality, and leadership. Effectively uses skills, cultural beliefs, and values of others for consultation/supervision. Brings out the best in others.	

Specific comments recognizing excellent performance or areas for improvement in interpersonal and communication skills:

Professionalism

1	2	3	4	5	NA
Learning Behaviors					
Does not show evidence of reading. Fails to acknowledge errors or limits to knowledge. Poor response to constructive criticism.	Fails to seek supervision. Only partially responsive to feedback. May require reminders to seek information.	Works at expected level of independence. Completes reading assignments reliably. Recognizes own limits and errors. Seeks help when needed. Accepts feedback without defensiveness.	Demonstrates curiosity and eagerness to learn. Seeks additional reading. Seeks out and responds to feedback.	Exemplary drive to learn. Demonstrates regular habits of self-directed learning. Goes out of his or her way to help others learn.	

Specific comments recognizing excellent performance or areas for improvement in professionalism:

Practice-Based Learning and Improvement

1	2	3	4	5	NA
Fails to perform self-evaluation. Poor understanding and application of principles of evidence-based practice (EBP). Resists or ignores feedback. Passive or negative participant in seminars.	Weak evidence of self-directed learning. Limited use of EBP skills in patient care.	Shows a growing habit of self-assessment and disciplined self-directed learning. Shows at least novice-level information-searching and EBP skills. Accepts feedback without defensiveness and uses it for change.	Committed to learning excellence. Seeks out and consistently incorporates feedback into improvement. Demonstrates regular, disciplined self-directed learning. Has expanded EBP skills.	Constantly evaluates and improves the effectiveness of own performance. Shows high level of initiative, eagerness, and success in self-directed, EBP learning. Positive participant or leader in seminars and rounds.	

Specific comments recognizing excellent performance or areas for improvement in practice-based learning and improvement:

Systems-Based Practice

1	2	3	4	5	NA
Unable to access or mobilize outside resources, especially systems that cater to patient's sociocultural background. Actively resists efforts to improve systems of care.	Significant weaknesses in ability to adapt treatment to the available sociocultural resources for the patient.	Appreciates organization of mental health systems that serve specific ethnic or sociocultural groups. Plans individual patient care accordingly. Advocates for quality culturally sensitive patient care. Assists patients in dealing with system complexities.	Shows initiative in assisting patients with proper resources and guiding them through the system.	Sophisticated understanding of sociocultural factors in mental health care systems. Develops elegant and imaginative strategies to maximize care. May be active as an advocate in mental health policy or community service.	

Specific comments recognizing excellent performance or areas for improvement in systems-based practice:

Estimation of how many patients this evaluation was based on: _____

Estimation of direct supervision hours: _____

Methods of evaluation include: ___ Chart stimulated recall ___ Case discussion or report ___ Patient care observation

Other supporting records: _____

Overall comments:

Overall Competence

Based on the level of skill expected from the satisfactory resident at this stage of training:

Unsatisfactory	Marginal	Satisfactory	Excellent	Exemplary
1	2	3	4	5

The resident met the goals and objectives of the clinical site/rotation. __ Yes __ No
If no, please explain in overall comments section.

This evaluation has been discussed and reviewed with the resident. __ Yes __ No

_____   _____
Resident Signature   Date

_____   _____
Supervisor Signature   Date

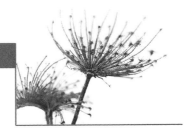

CHAPTER 3

Migration, Acculturation, and Mental Health

Carl I. Cohen, M.D.

Pachida Lo, M.D.

Carine Nzodom, M.D.

Samra Sahlu, M.D.

Learning Objectives

Examine the sociodemographics of the older immigrant population.

Consider several theoretical frameworks for understanding the migratory experience in older adults.

Explore various psychosocial factors that are associated with psychological risk in aging immigrants.

Review guidelines for the evaluation and care of older immigrants.

There are nearly 6 million elderly immigrants in the United States who are virtually invisible to the broader society (Zong and Batalova 2016). Most arrived earlier in life and have aged within their communities. A smaller number came later in life and have become valuable members of immigrant households. Treas (2008–2009) pointedly observed that nobody worries that elderly immigrants will take their jobs or join criminal gangs, and researchers largely neglect them, preferring to focus on working-age immigrants and their families. The overall aim of this chapter is to shed some light on the older immigrant population and their vulnerabilities with respect to psychological distress.

Basic Concepts

Migration

Migration refers to "the change in location of place of residence for an individual for any length of time" (Bhugra and Gupta 2011, p. 1). It can be within the boundaries of a country or from another country. Although the focus of this chapter is on transnational migration because of its more compelling cultural impact on the migrants, the United States has had several important internal migrations that had cultural importance as well. For example, in the Great Migration (1916–1930), 1.4 million African Americans left Southern states and migrated to Northern states, and in the westward expansion during the nineteenth century, waves of people moved across the country from Midwest states.

People migrate on the basis of *push* or *pull* factors. The former refers to political or social upheavals that may force persons to leave their homes, whereas the latter refers to factors that attract persons to a new place, such as hopes for a better economic life (Rack 1982). Bhugra and Gupta (2011) have identified three distinct but sometimes overlapping stages of migration: 1) a premigration stage, which involves the decision and preparation to migrate; 2) the migration process, which involves actual physical relocation; and 3) the postmigration stage or period of adjustment to the new home. During the first stage of migration, there are relatively lower rates of mental illness and health problems because of the typically younger age of immigrants at that stage, whereas problems with acculturation and the potential discrepancy between attainment of goals and actual achievement may emerge in the later stages.

Acculturation

The concept of *acculturation* is critical to understanding the migration process. Acculturation refers to "the dual process of cultural and psychological change that takes place as a result of contact between two or more cultural groups and their individual members" (Berry 2005, p. 698). Acculturation can occur as a result of migration, military invasions, or colonization. At the group level, acculturation involves changes in social structures, institutions, and cultural practices. At the individual level, it involves alterations in a person's attitudes and behaviors (Berry 2005). There are large group and individual differences in the ways in which people seek to go about their acculturation, and there may be differences within families that may engender conflict and stress.

Definition of Aging

The definition of aging itself varies cross-culturally and is relevant to how older migrants may perceive themselves and others. A review by Glascock and Feinman (1981) found that in non-Western traditional societies there are three ways to identify old age: change in social or economic role, chronology, and change in physical characteristics. Changes in social and economic roles had been the most common way to demarcate old age. However, most societies have multiple definitions of old age, which adds complexity and some ambiguity to any categorization. Dramatic demographic changes occurring worldwide have resulted in many societies having to redefine old age, and the Western definitions of aging can have profound psychological and social impacts on older immigrants. In many Western societies, persons are taking longer to reach various adult life stages (e.g., career, marriage, parenthood) and are living to older ages. Some gerontologists are conceptualizing age on the basis of life expectancy (Sanderson and Scherbov 2008); thus, with increases in life span, 65 years can be viewed as "the new 50."

Related to the conceptualizations of aging, *survivor* effects must also be considered when comparing older persons in different cultural groups. Although all older persons are survivors, there is considerable difference between a 75-year-old in a developed nation where half the population lives to that age and a 75-year-old in a developing nation where the life expectancy is age 60. The latter individual may have exceptional physical and psychological traits versus his or countrymen. Thus, new immigrants who may be exceptional survivors in their own countries can be just average in their host country, although as described in the next section, their heartiness may confer advantages in longevity over time.

DEMOGRAPHICS OF MIGRATION

In 2014, 14% of all immigrants were 65 years or older, and more than one in eight U.S. adults age 65 and older was foreign born, a percentage that is expected to continue to grow (Zong and Batalova 2016). The U.S. elderly immigrant population rose from 2.7 million in 1990 to 5.9 million in 2014, a 120% increase in 24 years (Zong and Batalova 2016). One projection estimated that the number of U.S. immigrants age 65 and older will quadruple to more than 16 million by 2050 and will represent nearly one-fifth of the elderly population (Treas and Batalova 2007). There have been notable changes in the regions of origin of older immigrants, with Latin America (38%) now exceeding Asia (29%) and Europe (28%) (Wilmoth 2012). Although most older immigrants go to large cities, increasingly more are found in towns and rural areas.

The rapid growth of the U.S. immigrant population age 65 and older has been driven by the aging of the long-term foreign-born population and the recent migration of older adults as part of family reunification and refugee admissions (Leach 2009). One group, older immigrants who arrived as children or very young adults, are aging "in place," that is, growing old in the communities where they have lived for most of their lives (Wilmoth 2012). The challenges that they face in later life closely resemble those of their U.S.-born racial and ethnic counterparts. A second group of older migrants comprise those persons who arrived relatively later in life and who face considerably greater difficulties with respect to acculturation. Their lack of integration into their host country coupled with strong attachments to their countries of origin contribute to these elders' sense of not feeling fully at home and aging "out of place" (Nesteruk and Price 2015).

A third group, the most numerous group of foreign-born elders, are those who came to the United States as young and early middle–age adults seeking educational and vocational opportunities. These immigrants spent their formative years in their countries of origin, and consequently, their socialization and basic education took place in sociocultural contexts different from those of the United States. However, they spent much of their working lives and raised their children in this country. Although they are long-term residents of the United States, they often maintain varying degrees of attachment to their countries of origin (Bhattacharya and Shibusawa 2009; Nesteruk and Price 2015; Wilmoth 2012).

In 2010, 60% of immigrants age 65 and older had entered the United States more than 40 years ago, and about 10% had been in the country fewer than 10 years (Wilmoth 2012). Among the latter, most were sponsored by their adult children whose immigration to the United States had preceded them. This has been facilitated by an immigration policy that began in 1965 under the Family Reunification Program, which gave naturalized U.S. citizens the opportunity to petition for their parents' entry outside the usual quota restrictions. Thus, the annual number of late-life immigrants (age 60 and older) admitted to the United States is roughly double the number it was in 1986, when it was 40,000 (Wilmoth 2012).

Late-life immigrants encounter many challenges versus immigrants who came earlier in life. These challenges include impaired physical health and financial and social barriers, such as difficulty obtaining some types of public assistance (especially following welfare and Social Security reform legislation in 1996), problems finding employment, language barriers and isolation caused by language difficulties (two-thirds of older immigrants do not speak English vs. one-third of immigrants under 60 years), and inability to drive or negotiate public transportation; a disproportionate number are female and poorly educated (Wilmoth 2012). These social disadvantages place late-life immigrants at risk for loneliness, dependency, and depression (Bhattacharya and Shibusawa 2009; Treas 2008–2009).

Compared with nonimmigrant older adults, elderly immigrants (especially those arriving in later life) are more likely to live in extended-family households (Wilmoth 2001). An extended-family household is defined as including at least one relative other than a spouse or a young child. Extended-family households can serve several purposes: 1) a pooling of resources in response to economic need; 2) a fulfilling of cultural practices of filial piety; 3) a way for the elderly person to perform housekeeping duties, cook, teach religious or cultural traditions, and provide care to grandchildren or other kin; and 4) a way to address problems of the aging person's health or social isolation. Gurak and Kritz (2010) found that about half of Indians, Filipinos, Vietnamese, Mexicans, and Dominicans lived in extended families, as opposed to about one in eight nonimmigrant white elders. On the other hand, elderly persons living in extended families have lower personal income and education, higher rates of physical disabilities, and lower levels of assimilation and English language skills.

Although foreign-born elderly generally have less personal income than U.S.-born elders, their family or household income is typically higher than that of U.S.-born elders. This reflects living arrangements (often with extended families) and proportionately high labor force participation by older men who have arrived within the past 10 years (Scommegna 2013). However, household income is unevenly distributed, with some groups, such as Filipino and Chinese immigrants, having high incomes, whereas Mexican immigrants have significantly lower household incomes versus their U.S.-born age peers. More recently, personal income has been declining vis-à-vis the nonimmigrant population because many new immigrants do not have the educational and professional skills of their predecessors. More elderly immigrants work in order to compensate for lower economic resources than do non-immigrants, and they also work to become eligible for Social Security and Medicare. Foreign-born elderly persons have poverty rates that are roughly twice the rate of U.S.-born elderly persons (16% vs. 8%), with poverty rates reaching 21% among elderly Latinos (Scommegna 2013).

Interestingly, foreign-born adults living in the United States are among the longest-lived older adults in the world when compared with nonimmigrant older adults in the United States and other industrialized countries. Additionally, among Medicare-eligible individuals, foreign-born U.S. blacks have the longest life expectancy of any group examined. This exceptional longevity stands in contrast to the well-documented disadvantages and correlated health risks among U.S.-born blacks (Scommegna 2013). This may reflect a high level of health on arrival, better health habits, a strong social network, and the return of some elderly immigrants to their native countries when they become older and more frail. Nevertheless, there are some ethnic elders who have higher rates of disability. For example, elderly Vietnamese have the highest rates of disability of any group, which was thought to reflect their arrival as impoverished refugees. Furthermore, some studies have found that these positive health factors diminish over time once immigrants' lifestyles converge with that of their surroundings (Lutsey et al. 2008). In particular, immigrants with low education are more susceptible to integrating U.S. diets and unhealthy lifestyle habits (Gallo et al. 2009), and health advantages disappear entirely within 15–20 years after migration (Abraído-Lanza et al. 2005).

THEORETICAL FRAMEWORKS

Life Course Perspective

Life course perspective refers to the study of people's lives (age-graded events and social roles); structural contexts; and social, cultural, and historical change (Elder 2001). Much of what are considered age effects in individuals and groups may be related not to the aging process but rather to the experiences of the cohort group to which the individuals belong. Individual trajectories interact with sociocultural processes. In societies undergoing rapid change, historical effects may take the form of a cohort effect, so various social changes distinguish the life experiences of successive cohorts (Elder 2001). Consider the potential psychological impact on elderly Chinese migrants to the United States of having lived through the warlord years, the occupation by the Japanese during World War II, the Communist Revolution, the Great Leap Forward and the ensuing famine, the Cultural Revolution, and the opening of the economy and market reform (Levkoff et al. 1995).

Nesteruk and Price (2015) argued that a life course perspective is a valuable tool for examining the complexities and diversities of elderly immigrants, especially with respect to such variables as an immigrant's country of origin, immigration history, age at immigration, timing of arrival, generational status, family constellation (e.g., underlying bonds and forces), available resources, and the area of settlement. The intersection of aging, immigration, and ethnicity can be explored more fully from the perspective of individual migrants and their familial ties, with particular emphasis on timing of immigration in the life course, sociocultural and historical contexts of sending and receiving countries, and length of residency in the host society.

Acculturation Model

In the previous subsection "Acculturation," we noted that acculturation occurs on several levels and entails both cultural and psychological change resulting from contact between two or more cultural groups and their members. On an individual level, this process can take years, manifesting in adaptations and behavioral changes in members of both groups (Berry 2005). Although the term itself is neutral, with respect to migration, patterns of dominance and nondominance emerge and result in one group undergoing more adaptation and change than the other (Berry 1997). Thus, migrant groups are viewed as the nondominant group and host communities as the dominant group, although individual- and group-level heterogeneity may exist (Berry 1970). The literature has tended to focus on the acculturation strategies of persons in the migrant group, but it is increasingly recognized that the dominant (host) group plays a powerful role in shaping acculturation.

There are a multitude of factors that contribute to individual heterogeneity, including baseline personality characteristics such as extraversion and self-efficacy (Berry 1970). The acculturation process itself is likewise affected by a variety of scenarios, both voluntary (immigration) and involuntary (forced displacement, colonization) (Berry 1997). The beliefs and attitudes held by the dominant group also affect the extent to which newcomers may integrate.

Berry (2005) has provided a useful model for understanding the various interactions between individuals or ethnocultural groups and the dominant larger society (Figure 3–1). The extent to which culture and identity are maintained can differ from older to younger migrants. The relationships sought by older migrants may be more along familial lines or within ethnic and religious communities, depending on the individuals and their circumstances. For example, older migrants who work outside the home may experience increased interfaces with larger society compared with those who live with their adult children and do not work.

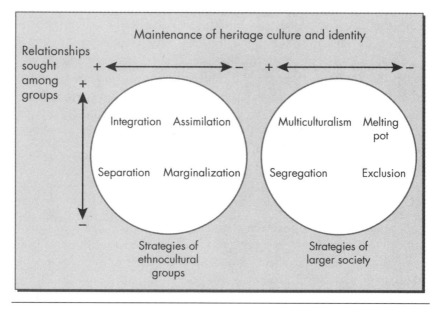

FIGURE 3–1.   Model of acculturation strategies of ethnocultural groups and the larger society.

Source.   Reprinted from *International Journal of Intercultural Relations*, Vol 29, John W. Berry, "Acculturation: living successfully in two cultures," page 705, Copyright (2005), with permission from Elsevier.

In Berry's acculturation model, from the point of view of nondominant groups (left side of figure), *assimilation* occurs when individuals do not wish to maintain their cultural identity and seek daily interaction with other cultures (i.e., they relinquish their heritage culture and become absorbed into the dominant society). On the opposite pole, *separation* occurs when individuals turn inward and place a value on holding onto their original culture and avoid interaction with the dominant culture. The hybrid strategy *integration* occurs when there is an interest in both maintaining one's heritage culture and participating in the larger social network. *Marginalization* occurs when there is little possibility of or interest in heritage cultural maintenance (often because of enforced cultural loss) and little interest in having relationships with people in the host culture (often because of exclusion or discrimination).

With respect to the dominant host culture (right side of figure), *melting pot* refers to assimilation sought by the dominant acculturating group. *Segregation* is separation forced by the dominant group. *Exclusion* is marginalization imposed by the dominant group. *Multiculturalism* is when the integration of diversity is an accepted feature of the society as a whole. Inconsistencies and conflicts between these various acculturation preferences are sources of difficulty for acculturating individuals. Generally, *acculturative stress* occurs when the acculturation experiences cause problems for acculturating individuals.

This model suggests that there must be reciprocal accommodation between the migrant and the host culture to facilitate various strategies. For example, for integration to occur, both groups must have positive attitudes toward multiculturalism and low levels of prejudice (Berry and Kalin 1995). On the opposite end, if the host culture promotes segregation or exclusion, it becomes difficult to attain assimilation or integration. From an individual perspective, the fewest attitudinal and behavioral changes result from the separation strategy, whereas the most changes occur with the assimilation strategy. Integration involves the selective adoption of new behaviors from the larger society and retention of valued features of one's heritage culture. Marginalization is often associated with major heritage culture loss and few ties to the dominant culture.

FACTORS INFLUENCING MENTAL HEALTH

Although the negative and disorienting features of immigration have been the focus of much research, for some groups, it is important to underscore that migration may be part of successful aging (Sokolovsky 2009). For example, coming to the United States and owning a home is considered an important achievement for many older immigrants. Like their younger counterparts, many older migrants can adapt their attitudes and behaviors to suit their new surroundings. It is the degree of adaptability that determines quality of life.

Sociodemographic, Biographical, and Societal Variables

Immigrants from another country may be from urban or rural areas and may come from different socioeconomic, cultural/ethnic, religious, and other backgrounds. Any of these variables can impact immigrants' adaptation to the host country. In addition, several immigration factors may affect adaptation to and mental well-being within the host culture. These include age at immigration; historical events leading to immigration; the degree of familiarity with cultural norms, laws, and institutions in the host country; and the presence of family, cultural, and religious institutions from the immigrant's background (Cohen et al. 2018). Relevant variables that have been associated with psychological distress among immigrants include older age, female gender, unemployment, lower education, widowhood or divorced marital status, poor language skills, chronic diseases, and lack of social support or living alone (Ebrahim 1992; Kirmayer et al. 2011).

Acculturative Stress

Applying the components of his acculturation model (see earlier subsection "Acculturation Model"), Berry (1997) reviewed studies of a broad age range of immigrants and found that with respect to acculturative stress, there are persuasive data indicating that the pursuit of integration is least stressful (especially where it is accommodated by the larger society) and that marginalization is the most stressful. The assimilation and separation strategies display intermediate levels of stress. This pattern of findings holds for various indicators of mental health. To what extent these patterns of acculturative stress apply to older migrants is unknown.

Distance From Immigration

Sakauye (2004) identified four subcategories of ethnic elders on the basis of distance from immigration and level of assimilation, each of which may be linked to specific psychiatric difficulties. The first group consists of immigrants who have arrived within the past 10 years, usually preceded by their children. Typically, they have language barriers and experience social isolation and cultural shock. Their mental health problems may include adjustment disorders or even posttraumatic stress disorder, and they may be more apt to display culture-bound syndromes.

A second group of immigrants are those who have been in the country for a decade or more. Many arrived when they were young adults, and their language skills are better. They may focus more on social and health-related issues.

Among native-born ethnic elders (usually second-generation immigrants), there are two categories. The first native-born group, poorly assimilated elderly persons, may encounter problems due to language barriers, poverty, fear of the majority group, social stressors, poor health, and inadequate health care. They also may present with culture-bound syndromes.

The second native-born group consists of those older adults who are generally well assimilated but who still feel the sociocultural impact of prejudice, discrimination, and even overt racism. Such individuals may have problems with self-esteem or difficulties concerning their racial or ethnic identity. They may feel socially isolated, depending on the demographics of their neighborhood.

Language Issues

As suggested in the previous subsection, language and culture congruity can substantially affect the mental health of immigrants. For example, a study in Canada found that immigrants who were neither francophone nor anglophone were more likely to report loneliness than those who were (De Jong Gierveld et al. 2015). Paradoxically, having a social network comprising predominantly speakers from their country of origin was associated with greater loneliness, perhaps because it limited the possibilities for broadening social contacts. On the other hand, a study in Hawaii found that the least culturally assimilated men of Japanese ancestry (95% U.S.-born) had the lowest prevalence of depressive symptoms, which might reflect cultural norms about reporting depressive symptoms or could indicate that individuals who identify as more Japanese have networks of extended family as typically seen in Japan, which can ameliorate depression (Harada et al. 2012).

Collectivism Versus Individualism

Collectivism and *individualism* are the two most widely used concepts in cross-cultural studies of stress and coping (Lee and Mason 2014). It is theorized that in more individualistic societies, such as Western Europe and the United States, that place more weight on individual rights, people are likely to control or change their environment to fit their own personal needs. By contrast, in more collectivistic societies that emphasize interdependence, such as those in East Asia, people are likely to cope by adjusting to group needs. However, among immigrant groups, these hypothesized differences may be modified by acculturation factors (Lee and Mason 2014). Bhugra et al. (2011) postulated that individuals who migrate from predominantly sociocentric or collectivist societies into a society that is predominantly egocentric or individualistic are likely to have problems adjusting to the new culture, especially if the migrant is sociocentric in his or her own belief system. An increase in ethnic density may help decrease distress that persons may be experiencing in adjusting to their new environment by providing a social support system. Thus, for an elderly migrant from Cambodia (a predominantly sociocentric society) to the United States (a predominantly egocentric society), her feelings of isolation and alienation may be attenuated if other people from Cambodia with sociocentric views surround her. On the other hand, as Bhugra et al. (2011) pointedly observed, persons from sociocentric societies who have an egocentric outlook may have minimal difficulties adapting to their host country.

Older adult immigrants may find themselves occupying comparatively lower social statuses. A shift in cultural context can result in a loss of status, felt particularly strongly in those whose cultures place a strong societal value on the role of elders (Ebrahim 1992). Vocational status can also place older individuals at higher risks for distress, particularly if their "departure status" is greater than their "entry status" (Berry 1997). Biological factors contributing to the mental health of older migrants include sequelae of sedentary lifestyles, dietary changes, and exposure to new diseases (Berry 1997). Moving to densely populated urban centers can amplify these effects. Lack of access to traditional healing practices can further isolate older adults from their cultures of origin.

Incongruence Between New Culture and Traditional Ethnic Responses

Sokolovsky (2009) has described how traditional ethnic responses can sometimes exacerbate difficulties. This is in part created by the modification in traditional roles that must be adapted to the exigencies of the new environment (Treas 2008–2009). For example, South Asian elders often reside with their daughters in the United States, whereas in India they would typically live with their sons. Some elders may move from one child to another over the course of several years. At the same time, authority and respect for elders become modified in a setting in which the elders have little financial capital, cannot speak the language, or cannot navigate around town. Although immigrant families tend to be *familistic* (having high kin togetherness and solidarity), the family ties create insularity and social isolation because older immigrants are often expected to care for grandchildren, prepare meals, and do housekeeping. They have little time for other activities and are trapped by linguistic limitations and lack of material resources, and they may lose access to the types of socially enmeshed neighborhoods that they had in their native country. With little control over these circumstances, many elders experience depression and loneliness (Treas 2008–2009). This may be more acute in women because among some immigrant populations, men will spend more time than women outside the ethnic family, and as a result, men typically have more extensive linkages to the broader community. Consequently, older men often have better mental health.

SPECIFIC IMMIGRANT GROUPS AND PSYCHOLOGICAL ISSUES

As noted in the preceding two subsections, there are a multitude of factors—attributable to both the individual and the host country—that contribute to mental distress among older immigrants. In this section, we describe some cultural patterns within various ethnic elder groups that might impact mental health. As always, it is important to avoid oversimplification and cultural stereotyping, and a person-specific approach is essential for good clinical care.

African Caribbean Elderly Immigrants

For African Caribbean immigrants, acculturation should be thought of as a tridimensional paradigm consisting of three relevant cultural dimensions: ethnic Caribbean culture, European American culture, and African American culture (Ferguson et al. 2012). Successful integration of these three cultural orientations may be advantageous for this population (Chen et al. 2008).

For African Caribbean immigrants, there is pressure not only to climb the middle-class ladder but also to become a black American, although this group has been one of the most oppressed groups in American history. These immigrants come primarily from countries where people of African descent are the majority population, and being grouped with the African American group leads to shock among many of them (Matthews and Mahoney 2005). Some older African Caribbean immigrants worry that their children will never move up to the middle class and become African American (Johnson 2007; Portes and Zhou 1993). Moreover, there is fear of downward assimilation into inner-city African American culture, which has been associated with poorer sociocultural adaptation and a predisposition to acquire a more defensive stance toward the white mainstream culture (Kasinitz et al. 2001; Portes and Zhou 1993; Waters 1999).

Latino Elderly Immigrants

In the United States, Latino immigrants are primarily from Mexico and Central America. Many of these immigrants have voluntarily entered the United States to seek employment and could be undocumented immigrants. However, some specific Central American immigrants (Nicaraguans, Guatemalans, and Salvadorans) migrated to the United States because of extreme political instability and have witnessed murder, rape, and torture or were themselves victims of political violence. Pine and Drachman (2005) noted that provisions are made for the health of refugee migrants but not for immigrants. The U.S. Congress passed the Personal Responsibility and Work Opportunity Reconciliation Act of 1996, which allows refugees to qualify for health services immediately, bypassing the 5-year minimum wait imposed on other immigrants (Singer 2004). Unfortunately, many Central Americans were not granted refugee or asylum status. Consequently, many elderly Latino immigrants may suffer from much lower access to health care.

Given that many Latino immigrants have a collectivist culture, they tend to settle in densely populated ethnic enclaves (e.g., Cubans in Miami); consequently, there is a higher retention of native culture and language and a diminished need to adopt the host culture (Rumbaut 1997). As these groups became more visible, other social groups began to feel more vulnerable, and social tension developed.

Although Latino immigrants help to meet local labor needs in many communities, their contributions are often overlooked. Instead, the emphasis is focused on their use of public spaces and local resources, which creates tensions in the community that affect the mental health of this group and hinders individuals' ability to enter the wider society (Sullivan 2006). Many Americans believe that undocumented immigrants wrongfully benefit from public services and do not contribute to society. These erroneous convictions have led to anti-immigration laws. For example, in 1994 in California, Proposition 187 attempted to bar undocumented immigrants from accessing health care, and in 2010, the state of Arizona passed an initiative to allow its law enforcement agents to question an individual's immigration status. The election of President Donald Trump in 2016 focused attention on Latino immigrants, and there is concern about the potential psychological impact of his policies. Immigrants may internalize the message that they are not wanted in the United States, which can contribute to or exacerbate mental health issues (Portes and Rumbaut 2001; Sullivan 2006).

Like Asian elder immigrants, Latino immigrants experience changing kin roles as other family members become more individualistic as part of assimilation with the host culture. This is in contrast to their native culture, which emphasizes a collective view of family, with elders commanding control and family providing a support system. This poses challenges to elderly Latino immigrants who live in enclaves and are less acculturated than other family members. Thus, paradoxically, a study in San Diego found that older Latinos living alone reported four times more extended kin than older whites, but many were less likely to turn to kin in times of need (i.e., they preferred to "suffer in silence") (Sokolovsky 2009).

Asian Elderly Immigrants

Asian elder immigrants are not a homogeneous group, and various Asian ethnic groups have different acculturation distress experiences. In particular, Japanese, Vietnamese, Chinese, and Indian immigrant elders have higher incidences of depression as compared with other community elderly populations (Gallo and Lebowitz 1999). Common acculturation stress factors include physical, psychological, financial, spiritual, social, language, and family adjustments.

Among Asian elder immigrants, their caregivers are increasingly removed from cultural norms of filial piety and parental authorities, and they place these elders in role transitions that are challenging during immigration (Ho et al. 2003; Lan 2002). The Asian elder may experience loss of power and respect because his or her role as cultural conservator and family decision maker may be undermined because of the disjunctions between expectations of family support and changing social reality. Asian elder immigrants may expect that their children will live with them or in closer proximity to provide support for them; however, having fewer accessible children may lead to the elder's sense of social isolation and insecurity.

Asian elder immigrants are more likely to have experienced war-related trauma or political turmoil in their early lives that affects their acculturation experience. For example, Japanese immigrant elders in the United States during and after World War II may have experienced prejudice, discrimination, and possibly forcible internment (Shibuswa and Mui 2001). Vietnamese and other Southeast Asians (such as Hmong and Laotian elders) may suffer from a higher degree of migration grief due to forced immigration as refugees after the Vietnam War (Ngo et al. 2001). As noted in the subsection "Life Course Perspective," elders from China likely experienced the Cultural Revolution and other political turmoil. Some elderly Indian and Pakistani immigrants experienced devastation from the loss of many lives during the riots relating to the partition of India (Bhardwaj et al. 2012).

Table 3-1 provides an overview of the acculturation processes found across various racial ethnic groups.

TABLE 3–1. Comparison of acculturation process across racial ethnic groups

	Acculturation characteristics
African Caribbean elders	Tridimensional acculturation paradigm Downward assimilation to African American culture
Latino elders	Undocumented immigrant status leading to reduced access to health care and other resources Slower process of acculturation due to collectivist culture
Asian elders	Conflicts between core cultural beliefs of filial responsibility and parental authority and Western focus on individuality Nonhomogeneous group with varying socioeconomic, war, and political experiences affecting acculturation

SPECIFIC MENTAL DISORDERS AMONG ELDERLY MIGRANTS

In determining the prevalence of mental disorders in immigrant groups, it is critical to recognize that prevalence of many common disorders varies cross-nationally and within nations, so the national, cultural, and sociodemographic backgrounds of the immigrant need to be considered.

Schizophrenia

There are compelling data that rates of schizophrenia are higher among immigrants versus people in the host population or in the immigrants' country of origin. However, there are little data specifically with respect to older adults, which is in part made more difficult by the low incidence rates of new-onset schizophrenia in later life. Moreover, diagnoses may be confounded by the clinician's lack of awareness of cultural norms. Because older persons are more apt than younger persons to subscribe to traditional beliefs and superstitions, it is likely that the prevalence of paranoid or psychotic ideation would be greater among elder immigrants (Yeo 2001).

A study in New York City documented very high levels of paranoid ideation or psychotic symptoms among blacks age 55 years and older, particularly among persons born in the Caribbean (Cohen et al. 2004). The investigators found that blacks were more than twice as likely as whites to experience paranoid ideation: 21% versus 9%. Within the black population, there were appreciable but statistically nonsignificant differences in the rates of expression of paranoid ideation or psychotic symptoms among U.S.-born blacks (18%), French Caribbean blacks (38%), and English Caribbean blacks (18%). Although paranoid ideation and/or psychotic symptoms were not associated with impaired daily functioning, there was a significant association with depressive symptoms.

Depression and Anxiety

Reported rates of depression and anxiety in immigrants have been inconsistent. Some studies showed that the rates of common mental disorders among migrants are higher than are those among members of the culture in their new country, but others showed either no difference or lower rates (Bhugra et al. 2011). In one of the more comprehensive studies, Aichberger et al. (2010) studied persons age 50 years and older in 11 European countries and found that first-generation migrants in northern and western Europe had higher rates of depression than did their indigenous age peers. Although migrants in southern Europe had higher rates of depression, these rates did not differ significantly from those of their indigenous age peers. Greater age, lower income, female gender, and physical illness contributed to depression.

Van der Wurff et al. (2004) postulated that depression risk for immigrants likely depends on the interplay of ethnicity, social class, and health factors. Moreover, rendering a diagnosis can be problematic because persons from traditional cultures typically express distress in somatic terms and their concepts of depression are different from those of the West; therefore, they may not differentiate among the emotions of anxiety, irritability, and depression (Bhugra and Mastrogianni 2004). It is important to be sensitive to the language of depression. For example, Bhugra et al. (1997) found that Punjabi women participating in a focus group in London recognized the English word "depression," but the older women used such terms as "weight on my heart/mind" or "pressure on the mind."

Suicide

Suicide rates vary considerably across immigrant groups, often reflecting cross-national differences. In the United States, suicide rates for African and Latino American elders are lower than that of whites, whereas rates among Japanese, Chinese, and Korean American elders are comparable to that of whites. Sakauye (2004) theorized that the lower rates of suicide found among some older ethnic minorities, despite their poverty or immigrant status, may reflect stronger family ties, the greater importance of elders in the minority family, and more powerful cultural or religious attitudes against suicide.

Posttraumatic Stress Disorder

Finally, some migrants are refugees from harsh political regimes, wars, and natural disasters, and the possibility of posttraumatic stress disorder should be considered. Note that posttraumatic stress may manifest in uncharacteristic ways. For example, Jenkins (1991) reported that Salvadoran refugee women in North America explained their suffering as *nervios*, a cultural category including dysphoria, aches and pains, and subjective bouts of feeling intense heat that are culturally created normative responses to abnormal stressors.

CLINICAL EVALUATION

One difficulty in the evaluation of older immigrants is the lack of valid diagnostic tools that recognize cultural and age differences in the expression of and coping with psychological distress (American Psychological Association 2013). Clinicians must critically examine assessment resources developed in a Western middle-class context before applying them to non-Western, non-middle-class participants. The World Health Organization has attempted to develop diagnostic instruments that are harmonious and consistent with the cultural, linguistic, and educational norms of specific subject populations (Jiang and Li 2016). Commonly used cognitive tests such as the Mini-Mental State Examination (Folstein et al. 1975) and the Montreal Cognitive Assessment (Nasreddine et al. 2005) are still prone to cultural and educational biases. Instrumental activities of daily living and everyday memory as a means to overcome cultural biases have been recommended instead by some gerontologists (Berry 2005).

In conducting a psychiatric assessment, clinicians rarely examine the elderly migrant's circumstances preceding, during, and after the migration. Bhugra and Gupta (2011) have proposed querying about premigration (e.g., reasons for migrating, preparations for emigration, whether the intention was to migrate singly or in a group, degree of control over the decision to migrate), migration (e.g., age and time since arrival, plans to return to or remain permanently in the new country, asylum status) and postmigration (e.g., aspirations and achievements, acculturation and adjustment, attitudes toward the new culture, support networks).

CLINICAL CARE

Ingleby (2011) has identified several elements that are necessary in adapting mental health services to the needs of migrants:

- Improving accessibility—Persons are entitled to receive mental health services and to have insurance to cover these services. For many older immigrants, these benefits are not available.
- Offering mental health services that draw from the individual's cultural heritage—These services should be provided in conjunction with services from the host country.
- Having professional interpreters—It is essential that professional interpreters be used as opposed to informal interpreters (e.g., kin, friends). Along with lack of accessibility, language barriers provide a major obstacle to obtaining services.
- Using *cultural mediators* or *brokers*—In many European countries, mediators are used to guide people to treatment, explain medical ideas, conduct outreach, and disseminate information.
- Using outreach and media to enhance health literacy (i.e., knowledge of the health system and the ability to make effective use of it)—Providers must be perceived as user- or migrant-friendly, and staff should receive training in cultural competency as it pertains to older adults.

Treatment of older immigrants can be challenging. Issues that may arise in therapeutic encounters include the following (American Psychological Association 2013; Bhugra and Gupta 2011; Mintzer and Faison 2009; Sadavoy and Lazarus 2004; Sakauye 2004; Yeo 2001):

- There may be issues related to authority figures; some people may expect more direction, whereas others may be more wary because of prior experiences of racism or sexual or physical violence.
- Patients may be overly deferential, inhibited, or ashamed of revealing personal feelings, or they may be hostile and suspicious.
- Persons who have not worked or who have lived in rural settings may have difficulties adhering to strict time appointments.

- For new immigrants, their primary psychological issues may revolve around adjustment issues, and they may be more apt to present with culture-bound syndromes, whereas more established immigrants may present with more social and health-related issues.
- There is often a need for bilingual therapists. Even established elderly immigrants may say that they cannot fully express their emotional state in English and that they can best express their thoughts when they revert to their language of origin. Language issues may become more pronounced among persons with dementia because language abilities typically decline during the course of the illness.
- Western biomedicine has its own culture (e.g., knowledge, beliefs, skills, values) based on scientific assumptions and processes that generate definitions and explanations of disease. Older patients who are familiar with other health traditions may rely more on such factors as nature, balance, or spiritual interventions to explain physical states.
- People may identify conditions that do not match those found in biomedical references, yet these conditions can have a direct impact on health care, adherence to recommended treatment, and full communication between patient and provider. Thus, culturally defined somatic disorders and culture-bound syndromes with their own beliefs about treatment may make the practice of culturally appropriate geriatric care more complex.
- Cognitive styles vary among cultures, so concepts of shame may be stronger than guilt, and clinicians must tailor their treatment accordingly.
- Contrasting values of independence versus community or family may result in conflicting expectations regarding the involvement of others in the provision of patient care.
- Involving family is often beneficial, especially among immigrants whose family may be their only social and emotional support.
- Clinicians should inquire about the use of indigenous healers and herbal remedies and the roles that faith, religion, and/or spirituality play in relieving the patient's symptoms.
- Group therapy may be useful for persons from sociocentric cultures, but this may raise issues of confidentiality and shame.
- In prescribing medications, clinicians should be aware that oxidative liver metabolism involving the cytochrome P450 enzymes is affected by both aging and ethnicity. There is considerable biodiversity involving the enzymes of the P450 system, so disproportionately more persons from certain ethnic groups may be more likely to be slow or fast metabolizers. In addition, dietary practices must be examined because some foods can affect drug metabolism.

- Therapists must ensure that patients do not take refuge in cultural differences to explain away all emotional reactions and behaviors.
- Clinicians should employ an ecological perspective to consider the ways in which each immigrant's unique set of characteristics interacts with the environment to place that person in varying positions of resilience or vulnerability.

KEY POINTS

- Despite comprising one-seventh of the immigrant population and nearly 5 million persons, elderly immigrants have been a largely invisible group to society and researchers.
- Immigration is a process, and the evaluation of an older immigrant must include an exploration of the periods prior to, during, and after immigration.
- Older immigrants can be best understood within a life course perspective that examines people's lives (age-graded events and social roles) within the context of social, cultural, and historical change.
- Acculturation involves the interaction of the individual migrant's behavior and attitudes toward the social structures and ideology of the host country. Stress can occur when the individual's style of acculturation is not accommodated by the host culture.
- Various factors impact the psychological well-being of older immigrants, including social class, gender, age at immigration, acculturation stress, level of assimilation, language abilities, and conflicts between traditional culture and adaptation to the host country.
- Rates of schizophrenia and psychoses seem to be higher among immigrants than among nonmigrants, although this disparity is less definitive among older immigrants. There are mixed findings regarding depression and suicide in older migrants, and rates of posttraumatic stress disorder are likely to be high among refugees.
- Clinical evaluation remains problematic because of the lack of valid culturally appropriate and age-appropriate diagnostic instruments.
- Clinical care should focus on enhancing accessibility, overcoming language barriers, integrating cultural heritage

and alternative health frameworks with the health and disease models of the host country, and using cultural mediators and more assimilated family members to assist with engagement with health and mental health systems.

QUESTIONS FOR FURTHER THOUGHT

1. Which of the following are the three distinct stages of migration as identified by Bhugra and colleagues?

   A. Decision and preparation to migrate, physical relocation, and postmigration.
   B. Precontemplation, decision and preparation to migrate, and physical relocation.
   C. Decision and preparation to migrate, physical relocation, and acculturation.
   D. Decision and preparation to migrate, postmigration state, and adaptation.

2. Which of the following stages of migration is associated with a relatively lower rate of mental illness and health problems?

   A. The migration process, involving actual physical relocation.
   B. The postmigration stage.
   C. The premigration stage.
   D. The precontemplation stage.

3. Which of the following is a challenge that late-life immigrants encounter versus immigrants who came earlier in life?

   A. Difficulty finding housing.
   B. Difficulty obtaining public assistance.
   C. Strenuous relationship with family members in the host country.
   D. Trouble communicating with loved ones in the country of birth.

4. Among Medicare-eligible foreign-born elders, which of the following groups has the longest life expectancy due to high level of health on arrival, better health habits, and a strong social network?

    A. Eastern Europeans.
    B. Filipinos.
    C. Blacks.
    D. Cambodians.
    E. Indians.

5. What is the dual process of cultural and psychological change that takes place as a result of contact between two or more cultural groups and their individual members called?

    A. Acculturation.
    B. Immigration.
    C. Migration.
    D. Colonization.

6. Match the following racial ethnic groups with the acculturation characteristics.

   1. African Caribbeans   2. Asians   3. Latinos

    A. Tridimensional acculturation paradigm.
    B. Downward assimilation to inner-city African American culture.
    C. Undocumented immigrant status, leading to reduced access to health care and other resources.
    D. Settling in dense population enclaves, which may slow the process of acculturation.
    E. Filial responsibility and parental authority core cultural beliefs that conflict with Western focus on individuality.
    F. Nonhomogeneous group with varying socioeconomic, war, and political experiences affecting acculturation.

7. Which mental disorder has a higher rate among immigrants, especially black immigrants?

    A. Bipolar disorder.
    B. Major depressive disorder.
    C. Schizophrenia and psychosis.
    D. Panic disorder.

8. A 62-year-old Japanese American male presents to the psychiatrist with his daughter for evaluation. The daughter states that the patient moved to the United States 2 months ago. He has

been irritable and complains of abdominal pain, knee pain, and headaches. He rarely smiles and constantly talks about his life back home. The patient does not speak English. Which measures should the psychiatrist take to ensure proper communication with the patient?

    A. Allow the daughter to translate during the evaluation because she knows the patient best.
    B. Bring in a nurse who reports that she speaks Japanese.
    C. Use a professional translation service and use terms referring to the patient specifically.
    D. Use Google Translate because it is the easiest way to obtain information.

9. During the evaluation of older immigrants, which tools best help the clinician perform a more thorough assessment as a means to overcome cultural biases?

    A. The Montreal Cognitive Assessment.
    B. The Mini-Mental State Examination.
    C. The Beck Depression Scale.
    D. Scales measuring instrumental activities of daily living and everyday memory.

10. Before prescribing a pharmacological agent to an elderly immigrant, it is most important that the clinician assess the use of indigenous healers, herbal remedies, the role of faith and religion, and which of the following?

    A. Cytochrome P450 enzymes.
    B. Patient's height.
    C. Patient's level of education.
    D. Patient's dentition.

SUGGESTED READINGS

Bhugra D, Gupta S, Bhui K, et al: WPA guidance on mental health and mental health care in migrants. World Psychiatry 10(1):2–10, 2011 21379345

Cohen CI, Elmouchtari M, Ahmed I: Working with elderly persons across cultures, in Transcultural Psychiatry, 2nd Edition. Edited by Bhugra D, Bhui K. London, Cambridge University Press, 2018, pp 552–569

Lewis-Fernández R, Aggarwal NK, Hinton L, et al (eds): DSM-5 Handbook on the Cultural Formulation Interview. Arlington, VA, American Psychiatric Association Publishing, 2016

Nesteruk O, Price CA: Long-term immigrants in middle and later life: changing views of home family. Sci Rev (Singap) 20(2):113–136, 2015

Sakauye K: Ethnocultural aspects of aging in mental health, in Comprehensive Textbook of Geriatric Psychiatry, 3rd Editon. Edited by Sadavoy J, Jarvik LF, Grossberg GT, et al. New York, WW Norton, 2004, pp 225–250

Treas J: Four myths about older adults in America's immigrant families. Generations 32:40–45, 2008–2009

REFERENCES

Abraído-Lanza AF, Chao MT, Flórez KR: Do healthy behaviors decline with greater acculturation? implications for the Latino mortality paradox. Soc Sci Med 61(6):1243–1255, 2005 15970234

Aichberger MC, Schouler-Ocak M, Mundt A, et al: Depression in middle-aged and older first-generation migrants in Europe: results from the Survey of Health, Ageing and Retirement in Europe (SHARE). Eur Psychiatry 25(8):468–475, 2010 20615669

American Psychological Association: Working With Immigrant-Origin Clients: An Update for Mental Health Professionals. Washington, DC, American Psychological Association, 2013

Berry JW: Marginality, stress and ethnic identification in an acculturated aboriginal community. J Cross Cult Psychol 1(3):239–252, 1970

Berry JW: Immigration, acculturation, and adaptation. J Appl Psychol 46(1):5–34, 1997

Berry JW: Acculturation: living successfully in two cultures. Int J Intercult Relat 29(6):697–712, 2005

Berry JW, Kalin R: Multicultural and ethnic attitudes in Canada: an overview of the 1991 National Survey. Can J Behav Sci 27(3):301–320, 1995

Bhardwaj U, Sharma V, George S, et al: Mental health risk assessment in a selected urban slum of Delhi: a survey report. J Nurs Sci Pract 1:1, 2012

Bhattacharya G, Shibusawa T: Experiences of aging among immigrants from India to the United States: social work practice in a global context. J Gerontol Soc Work 52(5):445–462, 2009 19585322

Bhugra D, Gupta S: Introduction: setting the scene, in Migration and Mental Health. Edited by Bhugra D, Gupta S. New York, Cambridge University Press, 2011, pp 1–14

Bhugra D, Mastrogianni A: Globalisation and mental disorders. Overview with relation to depression. Br J Psychiatry 184:10–20, 2004 14702222

Bhugra D, Gupta KR, Wright B: Depression in North India comparison of symptoms and life events with ocher patient groups. Int J Psychiatry Clin Pract 1(2):83–87, 1997 24936661

Bhugra D, Gupta S, Bhui K, et al: WPA guidance on mental health and mental health care in migrants. World Psychiatry 10(1):2–10, 2011 21379345

Chen SX, Benet-Martínez V, Harris Bond M: Bicultural identity, bilingualism, and psychological adjustment in multicultural societies: immigration-based and globalization-based acculturation. J Pers 76(4):803–838, 2008 18482355

Cohen CI, Magai C, Yaffee R, et al: Racial differences in paranoid ideation and psychoses in an older urban population. Am J Psychiatry 161(5):864–871, 2004 15121652

Cohen CI, Elmouchtari M, Ahmed I: Working with elderly persons across cultures, in Transcultural Psychiatry, 2nd Edition. Edited by Bhugra D, Bhui K. New York, Cambridge University Press, 2018

De Jong Gierveld J, Van der Pas S, Keating N: Loneliness of older immigrant groups in Canada: effects of ethnic-cultural background. J Cross Cult Gerontol 30(3):251–268, 2015 25982532

Ebrahim S: Social and medical problems of elderly migrants. Int Migr 30(s1):179–197, 1992

Elder GH: Life course, in The Encyclopedia of Aging, 3rd Edition. Edited by Maddox GL. New York, Springer, 2001, pp 593–596

Ferguson GM, Bornstein MH, Pottinger AM: Tridimensional acculturation and adaptation among Jamaican adolescent-mother dyads in the United States. Child Dev 83(5):1486–1493, 2012 22966917

Folstein MF, Folstein SE, McHugh PR: "Mini-mental state:" a practical method for grading the cognitive state of patients for the clinician. J Psychiatr Res 12(3):189–198, 1975 1202204

Gallo JJ, Lebowitz BD: The epidemiology of common late-life mental disorders in the community: themes for the new century. Psychiatr Serv 50(9):1158–1166, 1999 10478901

Gallo LC, de Los Monteros KE, Allison M, et al: Do socioeconomic gradients in subclinical atherosclerosis vary according to acculturation level? Analyses of Mexican-Americans in the multi-ethnic study of atherosclerosis. Psychosom Med 71(7):756–762, 2009 19661194

Glascock AP, Feinman SL: Social assets or social burden: treatment of the aged in non-industrial societies, in Dimensions: Aging, Culture, and Health. Edited by Fry C. Hadley, MA, Bergin & Garvey, 1981, pp 13–32

Gurak DT, Kritz MM: Elderly Asian and Hispanic foreign- and native-born living arrangements: accounting for differences. Res Aging 32(5):567–594, 2010 22984319

Harada N, Takeshita J, Ahmed I, et al: Does cultural assimilation influence prevalence and presentation of depressive symptoms in older Japanese American men? The Honolulu-Asia aging study. Am J Geriatr Psychiatry 20(4):337–345, 2012 21358388

Ho B, Friedland J, Rappolt S, et al: Caregiving for relatives with Alzheimer's disease: feelings of Chinese-Canadian women. J Aging Stud 17:301–321, 2003

Ingleby D: Adapting mental health services to the needs of migrants and ethnic minorities, in Migration and Mental Health. Edited by Bhugra D, Susham G. New York, Cambridge University Press, 2011, pp 231–244

Jenkins JH: The state construction of affect: political ethos and mental health among Salvadoran refugees. Cult Med Psychiatry 15(2):139–165, 1991 1874001

Jiang S, Li P: Current development in elderly comprehensive assessment and research methods. Biomed Res Int 2016:3528248, 2016 27042661

Johnson TP: Cultural-level influences on substance use and misuse. Subst Use Misuse 42(2–3):305–316, 2007 17558932

Kasinitz P, Battle J, Miyares I: Fade to black? The children of West Indian immigrants in southern Florida, in Ethnicities: Children of Immigrants in America. Edited by Rumbaut R, Portes A. Berkeley, University of California Press, 2001, pp 267–300

Kirmayer LJ, Narasiah L, Munoz M, et al; Canadian Collaboration for Immigrant and Refugee Health (CCIRH): Common mental health problems in immigrants and refugees: general approach in primary care. CMAJ 183(12):E959–E967, 2011 20603342

Lan PC: Subcontracting filial piety: elder care in ethnic Chinese immigrant families in California. J Fam Issues 23:812–835, 2002

Leach MA: America's older immigrants: a profile. Generations 32(4):34–39, 2009

Lee H, Mason D: Cultural and gender differences in coping strategies between Caucasian American and Korean American older people. J Cross Cult Gerontol 29(4):429–446, 2014 25260229

Levkoff SE, MacArthur IW, Bucknall J: Elderly mental health in the developing world. Soc Sci Med 41(7):983–1003, 1995 8545673

Lutsey PL, Diez Roux AV, Jacobs DR Jr, et al: Associations of acculturation and socioeconomic status with subclinical cardiovascular disease in the multiethnic study of atherosclerosis. Am J Public Health 98(11):1963–1970, 2008 18511718

Matthews L, Mahoney A: Facilitating a smooth transitional process for immigrant Caribbean children: the role of teachers, social workers, and related professional staff. J Ethn Cult Divers Soc Work 14:69–92, 2005

Mintzer J, Faison W: Minority and sociocultural issues, in Kaplan and Sadock's Comprehensive Textbook of Psychiatry, 9th Edition. Edited by Sadock BJ, Sadock VA, Ruiz P. Philadelphia, PA, Lippincott Williams & Wilkins, 2009, pp 4214–4224

Nasreddine ZS, Phillips NA, Bédirian V, et al: The Montreal Cognitive Assessment, MoCA: a brief screening tool for mild cognitive impairment. J Am Geriatr Soc 53(4):695–699, 2005 15817019

Nesteruk O, Price CA: Long-term immigrants in middle and later life: changing views of home family. Sci Rev (Singap) 20(2):113–136, 2015

Ngo D, Tran TV, Gibbons JL, et al: Acculturation, premigration, traumatic experiences, and depression among Vietnamese Americans. J Hum Behav Soc Environ 3:225–242, 2001

Pine BA, Drachman D: Effective child welfare practice with immigrant and refugee children and their families. Child Welfare 84(5):537–562, 2005 16435650

Portes A, Rumbaut RG: Legacies: The Story of the Immigrant Second Generation. Berkeley, University of California Press, 2001

Portes A, Zhou M: The new second generation: segmented assimilation and its variants. Ann Am Acad Pol Soc Sci 530:74–96, 1993

Rack P: Race, Culture, and Mental Disorder. London, Tavistock, 1982

Rumbaut RG: Assimilation and its discontents: between rhetoric and reality. Int Migr Rev 31(4):923–960, 1997 12293210

Sadavoy J, Lazarus LW: Individual therapy, in Comprehensive Textbook of Geriatric Psychiatry, 3rd Edition. Edited by Sadavoy J, Jarvik LF, Grossberg GT, et al. New York, WW Norton, 2004, pp 993–1022

Sakauye K: Ethnocultural aspects of aging in mental health, in Comprehensive Textbook of Geriatric Psychiatry, 3rd Edition. Edited by Sadavoy J, Jarvik LF, Grossberg GT, et al. New York, WW Norton, 2004, pp 225–250

Sanderson W, Scherbov S: Conventional and Prospective Measures of Population Aging, 1955, 2005, 2025, and 2045. Washington, DC. Population Reference Bureau, 2008. Available at: www.prb.org/excel08/age-aging_table.xls. Accessed December 7, 2017.

Scommegna P: Elderly Immigrants in the United States. Washington, DC. Population Reference Bureau, October 2013. Available at: www.prb.org/ Publications/Reports/2013/us-elderly-immigrants.aspx. Accessed December 7, 2017.

Shibuswa T, Mui A: Stress, coping, and depression among Japanese American elders. J Gerontol Soc Work 36:63–81, 2001

Singer A: Welfare reform and immigrants: a policy review, in Immigrants, Welfare Reform, and the Poverty of Policy. Edited by Kretsedemas P, Aparicio A. Westport, CT, Praeger, 2004 pp 21–34

Sokolovsky J: Ethnic elders and the limits of family support in a globalizing world, in The Cultural Context of Aging: Worldwide Perspectives, 3rd Edition. Edited by Sokolovsky J. Westport, CT, Praeger, 2009, pp 289–301

Sullivan TA: Demography, the demand for social services, and the potential for civic conflict, in Our Diverse Society: Race and Ethnicity—Implications for 21st Century American Society. Edited by Engstrom DW, Piedra LM. Washington, DC, NASW Press, 2006, pp 9–18

Treas J: Four myths about older adults in America's immigrant families. Generations 32:40–45, 2008–2009

Treas J, Batalova J: Older immigrants, in Social Structures: The Impact of Demographic Changes on the Well-Being of Older Persons. Edited by Warner S, Uhlenberg P. New York, Springer, 2007, pp 1–24

van der Wurff FB, Beekman AT, Dijkshoorn H, et al: Prevalence and risk-factors for depression in elderly Turkish and Moroccan migrants in the Netherlands. J Affect Disord 83(1):33–41, 2004 15546643

Waters MS: Black Identities: West Indian Immigrant Dreams and American Realities. Cambridge, MA, Havard University Press, 1999

Wilmoth JM: Living arrangements among older immigrants in the United States. Gerontologist 41(2):228–238, 2001 11327489

Wilmoth JM: A demographic profile of older immigrants in the United States. Public Policy and Aging Report. 22(2):8–11, 2012

Yeo G: Curriculum in Ethnogeriatrics. Stanford, CA, Stanford University Press, 2001

Zong J, Batalova J: Frequently Requested Statistics on Immigrants and Immigration in the United States. Washington, DC, Migration Policy Institute, April 14, 2016. Available at: www.migrationpolicy.org/article/frequently-requested-statistics-immigrants-and-immigration-united-states-5. Accessed December 7, 2017.

CHAPTER 4

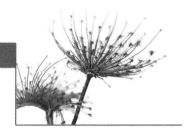

Asian Americans and Pacific Islanders

Madeline Nykamp

Shiv Lamba

Nhi-Ha Trinh, M.D., M.P.H.

Jai C. Gandhi, M.D.

Lan Chi Vo, M.D.

Iqbal Ahmed, M.D., FRCPsych

Learning Objectives

Describe the unique demographic characteristics of the elderly Asian American population in the United States.

Discuss the role of mental health stigma for this population.

List two or three alternative treatments this population will pursue in times of distress.

List and describe three idioms of distress unique to this population.

DEMOGRAPHICS

Asian Americans and Pacific Islanders (AAPIs) are the fastest growing population in the United States compared with any other racial group. In 2010 AAPIs represented 4.7% of the total U.S. population. According to a Pew Research Center analysis of 2010 U.S. Census Bureau data, the number of newly arrived Asian American immigrants (including those of mixed race) has surpassed the number of newly arrived Hispanic immigrants since at least 2009, with 36% of new immigrants coming from Asia versus 31% who were Hispanic. According to the U.S. Census Bureau, the population who reported being only Asian in race increased to 14.7 million in 2010 from 10.2 million in 2000, an increase of 46%. Of this 14.7 million, 9.6% were age 65 or older. According to the Administration on Aging, an agency of the U.S. Department of Health and Human Services, the number of Asians or Hawaiian and Pacific Islanders older than age 65 was 1.9 million in 2014 and is expected to grow to 2.5 million by 2020 and 7.6 million by 2050, from fewer than 1 million in 2000 (Pew Research Center 2012).

As a group, Asians come from diverse backgrounds and experiences and, in the United States, consist of the following subgroups: Chinese (22.84%), Asian Indian (19.46%), Filipino (17.40%), Vietnamese (10.67%), Korean (9.78%), Japanese (5.20%), and other Asian (15.04%) (Pew Research Center 2012). The term *Asian Americans and Pacific Islanders* encompasses a diverse ethnic and cultural realm. There are some 43 different ethnic groups—28 Asian and 15 Pacific Islander—who speak at least 32 primary languages and a host of dialects, many of which are not spoken outside their own communities. English proficiency varies according to the country of origin, level of education, and whether the person was born in the United States. According to the Pew Research Center (2012), when compared with all U.S. adults, Asian Americans have higher percentages of having a college degree (49% vs. 28%), higher median annual household income ($66,000 vs. $49,800), and greater median household wealth ($83,500 vs. $68,529).

According to the same analysis, however, differences in education and socioeconomic status exist among AAPI subgroups. Indian Americans lead all other groups by a significant margin in their levels of income and education. Seven in 10 Indian American adults age 25 and older have a college degree, compared with about half of Americans of Korean, Chinese, Filipino, and Japanese ancestry and about a quarter of Vietnamese Americans. Americans of Indian, Japanese, and Filipino origins have lower rates of poverty when compared with the general population. Conversely, Americans of Korean, Vietnamese, Chinese, and "other Asian" descent have higher poverty rates. The "other Asian" group represents 1.9 million adults and in the 2010 Census numbered more than 100,000 people, primarily Hmong, Laotians, Pakistanis, Bangladeshis, Burmese, Cambodians, and Thais. Although variations exist, in general, these subgroups are younger and have higher poverty levels (nearly 17%) than other Asian groups (Pew Research Center 2012).

The religious identities of Asian Americans are also quite varied. According to the Pew Research survey, about half of Chinese report no religious affiliation, most Filipinos are Catholic, about half of Indians are Hindu, most Koreans are Protestant, and a plurality of Vietnamese are Buddhist (Pew Research Center 2012). Overall, 39% of Asian Americans say religion is very important in their lives, compared with 58% of the U.S. general public.

Geographic settlement patterns differ as well. More than 70% of Japanese and two-thirds of Filipinos live in the West, compared with fewer than half of Chinese, Vietnamese, and Koreans and only about a quarter of Indians. Last, their pathways into the United States are very different and may, in part, contribute to socioeconomic status. About half of all Korean and Indian immigrants who received green cards in 2011 got them on the basis of employer sponsorship, compared with about a third of Japanese, a fifth of Chinese, one in eight Filipinos, and just 1% of Vietnamese. The Vietnamese are the only major subgroup to have come to the United States in large numbers as political refugees; the others say they have come mostly for economic, educational, and family reasons (Pew Research Center 2012).

CONCERNS OF THE ELDERLY AND THE ASIAN FAMILY

Asian families place a high value on the family and community. In most Asian families, there is a mutual interdependence among generations. Parents care for their children with the expectation that when they become old, their children will take care of them. This is a very different view from that of most American elders, who take pride in their independence and insist on not being a burden to their children. Most Asian families do not consider caring for the elderly a burden. In contrast to frail American parents who usually move in with their children, adult Asian children often live with their parents. In many traditional Chinese families, elders maintain full authority and financial control over the households of all their children, whether the children live with them or not. The eldest male, usually the grandfather, father, uncle, or eldest son, is the decision maker, although in some cases, the leader may be an older female. Psychiatrists need to identify and respect the family's hierarchy when treating any of the family members.

Asian elderly are often forced to deal with the stresses of divergent family and cultural values as well as the challenges of migration to a new country. Many move to the United States in their later years to be with their children, causing a harsh disruption to their expected life cycles. They can sometimes experience an uneasy role reversal: in the United States, the children have power because they speak English, and the elderly are dependent on them. It is far easier to age gracefully in a familiar society that values and highly respects the elderly, as most Asian societies do, than in a Western society that values youth and individualism over aging.

This disruption in the life cycle places Asian American elders at higher risk for mental health problems. However, they are more likely to underuse services because of the stigma attached to mental illness, as well as language barriers, social isolation, and limited access to services. Those who emigrated at younger ages have a better chance of adapting to new roles as their lives progress, and with assimilation and acculturation, they are more likely to access services (Kao and Lam 1997).

Multigenerational families—those with two or more adult generations (or a grandchild and grandparent) living under one roof—are more commonly seen in households headed by Asian Americans than those headed by a member of other racial and ethnic groups. Asian Americans are twice as likely as whites to live in households with at least two adult generations. Multigenerational homes in 2010 accounted for more than a quarter (28%) of all people living in households headed by non-Hispanic Asians compared with households headed by non-Hispanic blacks (26%), Hispanics (25%), and non-Hispanic whites (14%). The likelihood of multigenerational living varies markedly by Asian American group. Residents of households headed by someone who is Vietnamese (34%) or Filipino (33%) are most likely to be in multigenerational families, whereas those in households headed by Korean (20%) or Japanese (18%) persons are least likely to be in multigenerational families (Pew Research Center 2012).

In a country that is growing older and more diverse, elder care issues have particular resonance for many Asian Americans. Asian Americans older than age 50 are expected to grow from 4.3 million to 13.2 million over the next 40 years. According to a new study released by AARP, when compared with the general U.S. population of the same age, more Asian Americans 65 and older are on food stamps (14% vs. 9%), more are living at or below the poverty level (13% vs. 9%), and fewer have pensions or retirement accounts to draw on (22% vs. 37%) (Montenegro 2015). Those numbers often are masked by the broader segment of Asian Americans age 50 and older who live in a single household with other income-earning individuals, thus boosting the group's spending power to $60,466, the highest in the nation.

BELIEFS REGARDING ILLNESS GENERALLY AND MENTAL ILLNESS SPECIFICALLY

An individual's way of understanding the world can influence deci-sion-making processes regarding health care (Kelley 1973). Beliefs formed from individual ethnic identities can influence how one under-stands health and mental illness (Helman 1990; Vaughn et al. 2009). Many elderly Asian Americans bring to their understanding of health and illness a holistic view in which mind and body are more integrally connected than in Western systems, in which they are traditionally viewed as separate and distinct. A variety of medical systems exist in Asia, including complementary or alternative medicine (CAM) orienta-tions. In this section, we describe two examples of CAM, traditional Chinese medicine (TCM) and Ayurveda, to highlight how some older Asian American patients view health, illness, and treatment.

Older East Asian Americans subscribe to traditional Eastern philoso-phies such as Confucianism and Taoism that systematically address ail-ments as imbalances in life energy (or *qi*). These philosophies in turn influence a belief in a holistic view of the mind and body as being con-nected, which is reflected in TCM practices. Practiced on the body via acu-puncture, herbal medicine, and other physical treatments (e.g., massage), TCM is conceptualized as balancing the flow of vital energy to address ill-ness conditions (Kuriyama 2002). Stemming from this conceptualization, TCM makes little to no distinction between the cause and treatment of physical and psychiatric illnesses as Western medicine does (Liu 1981).

Ayurveda, roughly translated as "the science of life," is a complex medical system that emphasizes physical, mental, and spiritual health. Ayurveda classifies patients by body types, or *prakruti*, which are deter-mined by proportions of the three body humors, or *doshas* (Chopra 2017). Contrary to the scientific understanding of germs, viruses, and genetics, illness and disease are considered to be a matter of imbalance in the *doshas*. Disease is caused by an imbalance of the bodily humors and is cured by a restoration of the balance through meditation, diet, and natural medicine. Thus, the focus is on prevention and the use of herbal remedies to cure illness. Root causes for diseases are considered to include physical ailments, stress, and karma. Treatment for illness mostly involves changes in diet, herbal remedies, massage, application of oil to key areas, and rest.

CULTURAL BELIEFS REGARDING MENTAL ILLNESS

Asian Americans generally endorse more stigma associated with mental illness, including major depression, than do non-Latino whites (Georg Hsu et al. 2008). As a group, older Asian Americans may focus on psychosocial issues as the cause of mental illness (Jimenez et al. 2012). In the Primary Care Research in Substance Abuse and Mental Health for the Elderly (PRISM-E) study, a greater proportion of Asian Americans than non-Latino whites believed that family issues, medical illness, and cultural differences are main causes of mental illness. The authors of this study hypothesized that elderly Asian Americans are less likely to report distress in psychological terms and instead are more likely to report it through somatic symptoms. The expression of psychiatric problems through physical symptoms may be more congruent with Asian American cultural beliefs regarding the mind-body connection (Parker et al. 2001). For instance, as compared with their Western counterparts, depressed patients of East Asian and South Asian cultural origin tend to emphasize somatic rather than psychological symptoms and favor interpersonal or contextual rather than biological explanations for their distress (Ekanayake et al. 2012; Karasz 2005; Karasz et al. 2007; Kleinman 1977; Yeung and Kam 2005).

Similarly, in a study of illness beliefs in depressed Asian Americans by Chen et al. (2015), most subjects in the study (68.5%) identified a psychological stress as the most likely cause of their problem, with a romantic relationship or marriage the most commonly cited psychological stress (24.7% of the total), followed by work or job problems (14.7%) and problems with family relationships other than with a spouse (11.6%). Significant minorities of subjects reported a belief in medical (19.5%) or psychological (16.8%) causes. When combined, relationship-based stresses (including marital stress, other household relationships, in-laws, and unspecified interpersonal conflicts) accounted for 40.6% of all responses. This high proportion is consistent with a known emphasis in Chinese populations on strong social networks, particularly within a caregiving context (Aranda and Knight 1997; Cheng et al. 2013).

Finally, in a qualitative study focusing on attributions of mental health disorders, Asian American respondents were more likely to provide attributions that normalized the behaviors, that is, to attribute mental health problems to normal behavior (e.g., "he's just getting old") (Bignall et al. 2015). The authors of this study hypothesized that the tendency to normalize may be explained by the large amount of stigma associated with mental illness in Asian American communities. This is related to the principle of *saving face*, a core social value in many Asian cultures, which focuses on the avoidance of humiliation or embarrassment, maintaining dignity, and preserving one's reputation and the reputation of one's family. Many Asian Americans with mental disorders describe feelings of failure and shame when they are unable to meet the high expectations of their families (Lin 2013). Asian Americans have been described as less willing to speak to anyone about mental illness, perhaps because of mental illness being highly stigmatized and the need to preserve a sense of dignity (Sue et al. 2012). In Chen's study, nearly half of the depressed Asian Americans interviewed (40%) reported that they would conceal the name of their problem from everyone, with an additional 5.8% reporting that they would conceal it from all but a few trusted confidants. Similarly, although 32.6% identified the name of their problem (depression) as a mental disorder, only 8.9% reported they would use this terminology when discussing it with others (Chen et al. 2015).

CULTURAL BELIEFS REGARDING TREATMENT

Many elderly Asian Americans prefer to use alternative medical practices and self-care over professional treatment. In the Chen et al. (2015) study of depressed Asian Americans, the vast majority of subjects (75%) preferred nonmedical self-help or lay help methods for addressing their symptoms. In the PRISM-E study, there was no single treatment modality that Asian Americans preferred when compared with non-Latino whites, and as a group, Asian Americans reported being unwilling to speak to anyone if they had a mental health problem (Jimenez et al. 2012). Southeast Asian refugees tend to hold the belief that illnesses are inevitable in life, making them less likely to turn to Western medicine for treatment (Uba 1992).

This guarded approach to seeking treatment enhances the understanding of why Asian Americans report being unwilling to speak to others regarding mental health concerns. Asian Americans have been found as a group to be less likely to seek social support because they are more cautious about potentially disturbing their social network (Kim et al. 2006).

When they do seek mental health treatment, a number of Asian Americans will use CAM or visit a traditional healer before consulting a Western doctor (Feng et al. 2006; Lai and Chappell 2007). One community-based study that included Asians, Hispanics, and non-Hispanic whites showed that 47.8% of respondents reported using CAM over the past year (Najm et al. 2003). Dietary supplements (47.4%), chiropractic treatments (16.3%), home remedies (15.9%), acupuncture (15.1%), and Asian medicine (12.8%) were the most frequently cited therapies. The majority of CAM users (62.4%) did not inform their physicians that they were using these therapies, but 58% consulted their physician for the same problem for which they used CAM. Asians were more likely to use CAM when pain was the complaint, which is also important to note because of the high degree of somatization associated with mental illness in this population.

Because TCM practitioners are often the first health practitioners contacted for treatment of illness among Chinese immigrants (Lin 1983), such healers might act as the sole provider or as gatekeepers in this community. Understanding the factors that determine TCM use becomes especially important in the context of psychiatric service utilization because reliance on TCM has been suggested as a reason for this group's consistent underuse of and delay in accessing Western psychiatric services (U.S Department of Health and Human Services 2001). Asian Americans, females in particular, are also more likely to rely on religious services, elders, or ethnic and cultural organizations for mental health treatment, and they might even perceive seeking treatment outside of the family as shameful (Xu et al. 2011).

The influence of Confucianism and the hierarchical nature of many Asian cultures stress respect for authority figures, including therapists. Therefore, patients who present for treatment may not voice objections to treatment plans during sessions but later may fail to implement them if they do not agree with the therapist's recommendations. The provider should not assume that recommendations are being followed and should check in periodically with the patient in a nonconfrontational manner to ensure that the patient is following the treatment recommendations.

Understanding Patient Health Beliefs

By understanding Asian American patients' beliefs about the causes of mental illness in general and the shame and stigma that have been linked to mental health help seeking and recovery in this population, providers can better tailor treatment plans to Asian American patients in a culturally sensitive manner. Kleinman et al. (1978) first described a method to understand a patient's explanatory model, which can be very helpful when eliciting a history and attempting to negotiate a treatment plan. In using this method, the provider asks the following questions:

- What do you call your problem?
- What causes your problem?
- Why do you think it started when it did?
- How does it work—what is going on in your body?
- What kind of treatment do you think would be best for this problem?
- How has this problem affected your life?
- What frightens or concerns you most about this problem and treatment?

In addition, given the important role of CAM in this patient population and the likelihood that the patient may not volunteer information on his or her use of CAM, the provider should always ask about past and current use of traditional and alternative healing to understand and respect the patient's choices. DSM-5 now includes an Outline for Cultural Formulation and a Cultural Formulation Interview to aid providers in conceptualizing an individual patient's explanatory model of illness and in working with the patient to understand which treatment options are acceptable to him or her (American Psychiatric Association 2013).

Psychiatric Disorders Among Asian Americans

As a group, elderly Asians living in the United States have the lowest lifetime prevalence of any psychiatric disorder (14.6%) when compared with respondents from other minority and non-Latino white groups (range 17.3%–26.8%), and this was found to be statistically significant (Jimenez et al. 2010). However, the state of Asian American mental health is difficult to summarize with statements about prevalence of mental disorders compared with those of other groups because there has been limited consistency of findings due to variability in the methodologies used to identify psychological distress and syndromes; type of clinical problem; Asian American subgroup considered; and other variables such as acculturation, gender, and age. Further, a relatively small amount of research has been dedicated to examining psychiatric illness in these populations specifically, and even less has been conducted regarding mental health issues in older AAPI populations.

An added historical challenge in reviewing psychiatric disorders in AAPI populations is the low level of response from these communities to surveys assessing problems across a population (Whaley 1997). Asian Americans in general, and Korean Americans in particular, are more prone to premature termination of psychiatric care because of cultural and social pressure to solve mental health issues in other, more traditional ways (Lee et al. 2014). Because so little is known, it can be difficult for clinicians to find distinct, culturally competent guidelines for the management of psychiatric disorders in the AAPI population. In this section, we describe the available data.

Substance Use Disorders

Older Asians exhibit statistically lower lifetime prevalence rates of any substance use disorder and alcohol abuse and dependence. Comorbid substance use disorders in older Asian Americans are consistently found to be rare, but Pacific Islanders and Native Hawaiians are both more likely to suffer from substance use disorders than are Asian Americans. In Asian Americans, Pacific Islanders, and Native Hawaiians, males are more likely than females to have substance abuse issues across all age groups (Wu et al. 2013).

Depressive Disorders

Prevalence rates for depression vary greatly, depending on evaluation method chosen, AAPI subgroup studied, country of origin, and duration of time in the United States, making it difficult to determine prevalence rates. The National Latino and Asian American Study found that 9.1% of Asian Americans endorsed an affective disorder. This study sampled Filipinos, Vietnamese, Chinese, and "other" Asians. Compared with other racial and ethnic groups, Asians still had the lowest rates of lifetime major depression, and Filipinos had the lowest rate within the Asian group (Jackson et al. 2011). Among older U.S. Asians, Jimenez et al. (2010) found the lifetime prevalence of any depressive disorder to be 7.7% (rates for major depressive disorder and dysthymia were 7.5% and 2.4%, respectively). Higher rates of psychopathology were found in older Asian immigrants compared with Asians born in the United States. Jimenez et al. (2010) found that most Asian immigrants who were depressed had poorer English fluency. It was postulated that this may have increased their sense of social isolation, thus increasing anxiety and depression and limiting access to mental health services.

Very little is known about the prevalence rates of depressive disorders among Indians in the United States, although several large epidemiological studies have been conducted in India. A large study recently published by the World Health Organization found 12-month prevalence rates of mild, moderate, and severe depression among older Indians (age 50 and older) to be 13.6%, 12.4%, and 8.2%, respectively (Kulkarni and Shinde 2015). Similarly, little is known about rates of depression among elderly Korean Americans. Studies from South Korea have found prevalence rates of elderly major depression to vary between 4.2% and 7.3%, with variability thought to be due to diagnostic tool used (Cho et al. 2011).

Depression has variable presentations due to cultural differences and attitudes toward mental illness. Depressed Chinese American adults in one study initially presented to their primary care physician with somatic symptoms, including fatigue, insomnia, and headache. Those experiencing somatoform disorders were generally much more likely to seek medical help (Kung and Lu 2008). These findings are consistent with those of several other studies (Cheng 1989; Kirmayer and Robbins 1996; Kleinman 1980). Jenkins et al. (1990) pointed to cross-cultural differences in the definition of selfhood as a possible reason for the differences in reporting depressive symptoms.

Another issue is health literacy regarding depression and mental illness. Among Chinese American adults, more than half of the depressed patients answered "I don't know" when asked what their condition was called. Most were unaware they had any psychiatric problems. After an official diagnosis, nearly half stated they had never heard of major depressive disorder (Kung and Lu 2008; Yeung et al. 2004). This suggests that psychoeducation is an extremely critical component of the management of depressive disorders in this population.

Posttraumatic Stress Disorder

Posttraumatic stress disorder (PTSD) is prevalent among older adults from Vietnam and Cambodia (Hinton et al. 1993; Tran et al. 2010). These individuals were exposed to trauma, near death due to starvation, and squalid conditions in refugee camps and have difficulties in acculturation and adaptation. High rates of PTSD (up to 62%) have been reported among Cambodian refugees, and PTSD and major depression were found to be highly comorbid in this group (Marshall et al. 2005). Panic attacks have also been reported in both Vietnamese and Cambodian refugees. Exposure to adverse race-related events in Pacific Islander veterans of the Vietnam War have been shown to have a significant impact on the development of PTSD and other psychiatric disorders (Loo et al. 2005). These adverse events include a sense of nonbelonging, an absence of bonding with their military comrades, suddenly having a crisis of basic belief and identity, the need to prove themselves, and eventual disillusionment with the war effort and their initial patriotism.

Schizophrenia and Psychotic Disorders

Prevalence data on schizophrenia and psychotic disorders in elderly AAPIs living in the United States are very limited. Studies from Asian countries have found lifetime prevalence rates of schizophrenia for older adults in the following subgroups: Chinese 0.19%–0.47% (Gee and Ishii 1997), Japanese 0.19%–1.97% (Gee and Ishii 1997), South Korean 0.34%–0.65% (Lee et al. 1990), and Indian 1.5% (Seby et al. 2011). Relatively little is known about inpatient psychiatric service usage by AAPIs when compared with other ethnic groups (Sentell et al. 2013).

Suicide

Research has demonstrated that elderly AAPI women are at higher risk for suicide relative to other minority groups within the same gender and age categories. According to the U.S. Department of Health and Human Services (2012), the completed suicide rates for AAPI women is almost twice that of other women in the same age group: 7.34 per 100,000 for AAPIs, 4.21 per 100,000 for non-Hispanic whites, 0.77 per 100,000 for African Americans, 1.03 per 100,000 for Latinos, and 0.00 per 100,000 for American Indians and Alaska Natives. Yang and Won-Pat-Borja (2006) performed a thorough literature review and concluded that elderly Asian women were at higher risk for suicide than elderly women in other groups. Furthermore, U.S.-born Asian women reported higher rates of suicidal ideation and suicide plans than U.S.-born Asian men and foreign-born Asian men and women (Duldulao et al. 2009). Bartels et al. (2002) examined suicidal and death ideation among older primary care patients with depression, anxiety, and at-risk drinking and found elderly Asian primary care patients to have the highest prevalence of suicidal or death ideation (56.8%) and elderly African American primary care patients to have the lowest prevalence (27.0%).

Similar findings have been seen in many Asian countries as well. Suicides among older South Koreans rose to 77 per 100,000 in 2009 (Park et al. 2016). In urban China, suicides among persons ages 70–74 increased to nearly 34 per 100,000 (Zhong et al. 2016), and the World Health Organization (2011) reported increasing suicide rates in Hong

Kong, Japan, Malaysia, and Singapore. Because of reporting variability, the rates may actually be underreported. Compared with rates in Western countries, suicide rates in Asian countries are generally higher, the male versus female differences are lower, and acute life stress (family conflicts, job and financial security) plays a more important role (Chen et al. 2012). Additional contributors are changes in traditional value systems, rapid economic changes, access to lethal means (e.g., pesticide poisoning, jumping), and sociocultural attitudes toward suicide.

Dementia

The incidence of dementia increases with increasing age, and racial and ethnic disparities in dementia incidence are known to exist in the United States. In fact, the *National Plan to Address Alzheimer's Disease* (U.S. Department of Health and Human Services 2017) and the Alzheimer's Disease–Related Dementias Conference road maps (Alzheimer's Association and Centers for Disease Control and Prevention 2013) have both identified the reduction of these disparities in dementia as national priorities. A recent study (Mayeda et al. 2016) conducted the first comparison of incidence rates among six minority groups in the United States. African Americans were found to have the highest incidence of dementia (26.6/1,000 person-years [PY]), followed by American Indians and Alaska Natives (22.2/1,000 PY). Intermediate incidence was identified for Latinos and Pacific Islanders (both at 19.6/1,000 PY), and the lowest incidence was for Asian Americans (15.2/1,000 PY).

Dementia caregiver burden is thought to be an acute reaction to providing care when a new need arises or existing demands intensify. Caregivers who are unable to adapt or modify strategies to meet these needs develop burden. Subsequently, to facilitate the development of appropriate interventions, it is important to understand how different cultures conceptualize dementia and ways to cope effectively. In India, for example, Hindi- and Punjabi-speaking caregivers perceive dementia as stemming from lack of effort by the person with dementia and lack of family care. Thus, an appropriate strategy would be to assist the person with dementia in addressing the problems, and some family involvement should be part of the plan (La Fontaine et al. 2007).

Other conceptualizations of dementia among Asian American caregivers include a biomedical model, a folk model, and a mixed-folk model (Chan 2010). In the biomedical model, caregivers refer to symptoms and diseases and use biomedical terms such as *Alzheimer's disease*. In the folk model, cognitive symptoms are seen as a "normal part of aging," and caregivers may use terms such as "confused" or may attribute memory loss to the patient's having a "difficult" personality and not being sufficiently "open-minded." In the mixed-folk model, biomedical terms are used, but dementia is thought to be due to psychosocial stress. In addition, some caregivers may see dementia as part of heaven's will, or *tian ming*, a Confucian concept that means to follow the nature of the universe. These beliefs can help caregivers accept the challenges of caregiving and avoid the guilt that is often seen in other groups.

PROTECTIVE AND RISK FACTORS

Traditionally, immigrants have lower rates of psychiatric illness than do U.S. natives, although this benefit is inversely related to the level of acculturation the immigrant achieves, and this protective factor often disappears with the next generation. However, it does suggest that elderly immigrants who have not acculturated within the United States may be somewhat protected against mental illness (Breslau et al. 2007). Chinese Americans who immigrated to the United States after age 18 are at a lower risk of depression, anxiety, and suicidal ideations than those who arrived before age 18 years. This might be due to younger immigrants having more opportunities to come across cultural conflicts (e.g., in school). Older immigrants might be more insulated from this conflict because they likely have already established their worldview and internal values (Zhang et al. 2013).

Some studies have shown that a stronger attachment to one's racial or ethnic group might be protective against psychiatric disorders. Additionally, fewer opportunities to participate in cultural activities or use one's native language are associated with an increased risk of psychopathology (Burnett-Zeigler et al. 2013). Among Chinese immigrants at senior centers, subjects who reported their health was good, lived with others, and reported being satisfied with aid from family members were least likely to endorse depressive symptoms (Mui 1996).

CULTURE-BOUND SYNDROMES AND UNIQUE PRESENTATIONS

Culture-bound syndromes are mental conditions or psychiatric syndromes whose occurrence or manifestations are closely related to cultural factors and thus warrant understanding and management from a cultural perspective. Approaches to culture-related specific syndromes have gone through several stages, reflecting the history of cultural psychiatry. The phenomena were initially called *peculiar psychiatric disorders* and later *culture-bound syndromes*. It is often argued that most such conditions are neither culture-bound (because of occurrence across many cultures) nor clearly syndromal (because of the variability in symptom presentations). DSM-IV-TR (American Psychiatric Association 2000) retained the latter terminology. By contrast, DSM-5 (American Psychiatric Association 2013) has redefined this category under *cultural concepts of distress* (Keshavan 2014). The number of culture-bound syndromes was expanded to 25 syndromes in DSM-IV-TR; this number was reduced to 9 in DSM-5. In DSM-IV-TR, 7 culture-bound syndromes were seen as recurrent, locality-specific patterns of aberrant behavior and troubling experiences that may or may not be linked to a particular DSM-IV diagnostic category (Ventriglio et al. 2016).

As a result of the reexamination of DSM-IV's glossary of culture-bound syndromes, the "boundedness" feature of the culture-bound syndromes was drastically challenged because its implication of uniqueness has been weakened by migrations and the subsequent broadening of geodemographic areas. Concepts of illness previously considered to be indigenous have been incorporated in contemporary descriptions (and vice versa). Instead, distress becomes the common conceptual umbrella for three more precise and useful concepts, referred to in DSM-5 as cultural concepts of distress.

Cultural concepts of distress refer to ways that cultural groups experience, understand, and communicate suffering, behavioral problems, or troubling thoughts and emotions. This distress becomes the common conceptual umbrella for three distinctive categories. The first category is *cultural syndromes*. These are entities characterized by clusters of co-occurring symptoms that may or may not be recognized as an illness within the culture. These conditions occur and are relevant in the societies of origin and may be noticed by an outside observer. DSM-5 includes nine of these conditions, adequately supported by research. The second category is *cultural idioms of distress*. These expressions are linguistic terms, phrases, or even colloquial ways of talking about suffering that are shared by people from the same culture. They are considered to be neither mental or emotional illnesses nor diagnostic categories. These idioms may include crying styles, body postures, and somatic manifestations that should be approached in a systematic, empirical way. The last category is *causal explanations*, a needed remnant of the rich explanatory models concept of Kleinman et al. (1978) (see section "Understanding Patient Health Beliefs"). These explanations convey deeply ingrained views and beliefs about what the patient and his or her family consider the etiology of the reported symptoms, illness, or distress. They can be part of folk classifications of disease used by lay-people or healers, but, beyond their formal presentation, they may also entail an anticipation of the patient's trust, faith, hopes, and expectations (Alarcón 2014; American Psychiatric Association 2013).

These concepts are discussed in the introductory chapter of DSM-5, and examples are provided in Section III and the appendix of DSM-5. These concepts suggest cultural ways of understanding and describing illness experiences that can be elicited in the clinical encounter. These concepts—syndromes, idioms, and explanations—are more relevant to clinical practice than the older formulation of culture-bound syndromes. They influence symptomatology, help seeking, clinical presentations, expectations of treatment, illness adaptation, and treatment response. The same cultural term often serves more than one of these functions.

Cultural Concepts of Distress

In Asia and among Asian refugees and immigrants, patients commonly present with anxiety that can be understood as one of various functional somatic syndromes. Some of these anxiety disorders could be considered as cultural concepts of distress, some as idioms of distress, and some as causal explanations. These distress syndromes often produce catastrophic cognitions about anxiety-type somatic and psychological symptoms. These functional somatic syndromes should be understood and specifically assessed and addressed in order to optimize the evaluation and treatment of anxiety disorders among Asian individuals (Hinton et al. 2009).

There are many weakness-related syndromes in Asia and among Asian refugees. Among Asian groups, many syndromes generate catastrophic ideas about energy depletion. Symptoms such as poor sleep and appetite, and worry itself, are particularly feared because they are thought to deplete the body. Asian patients often treat anxiety-type somatic and psychological complaints by taking medications that purportedly increase bodily energy, such as vitamin injections or other supplements. The clinician should address energy depletion–related fears (e.g., fear of "heart weakness") and frame proffered treatments (e.g., prescribed medications) as increasing mental and bodily energy directly by effects on nerve transmission and indirectly by improving sleep and appetite (which are key energy-restorative processes) and as decreasing worry (which is thought to be an energy-depleting process). An understanding of Asian distress syndromes is needed to design adequate assessment and treatment of anxiety disorders in these populations. The patient's concerns about anxiety symptoms—about having a "syndrome"—must be addressed to stop the vicious cycle of arousal, attention, and catastrophic cognitions. Explanatory models about anxiety symptoms that generate catastrophic cognitions reflect certain culturally determined meaning and significance of anxiety symptoms (Hinton et al. 2009).

Some of these explanatory models may be anxiogenic, and this will have a profound influence on the rates, chronicity, phenomenology, presentation, and self-treatment of anxiety disorders. These explanatory models may result in higher rates of certain kinds of anxiety-generating catastrophic cognitions about autonomic arousal symptoms. The clinician should elicit not only the patient's anxiety symptoms but also his or her symptom schemata, illness attributions, and illness representations—what the patient thinks the symptoms mean and their implications (Hinton et al. 2009).

Challenges in the Diagnosis and the Use of Cultural Concepts of Distress

The presence of cultural concepts of distress among Asian patients can have specific challenges for the clinician. For example, ambiguity in the meaning of the term *neurasthenia* in the past apparently has encouraged its inappropriate use. A number of patients diagnosed by Chinese psychiatrists as having neurasthenia (*shenjing shuairuo* in Mandarin Chinese) could be reclassified as having major depression (Lin and Cheung 1999).

Korean and Korean American patients experiencing similar mixtures of a wide variety of somatic and emotional symptoms often label themselves as suffering from *hwa-byung*, which literally means both "fire disease" and "anger disease." As these terms suggest, patients believe that their problems are caused by chronic unresolved anger, resulting in excessive accumulation of the fire element, as conceptualized in Asian medicine theories. This leads to an imbalance of the body. *Hwa-byung* is another example of how Asians conceptualize the body-mind relationship. Although the concept denotes the existence of chronic social stress as well as emotional responses, most patients with *hwa-byung* believe that their problems are primarily physical. Some are even convinced that the anger and the chronic imbalance have resulted in the accumulation of harmful substances in the epigastric area in the form of a mass that could kill them if untreated. This would be considered more of a cultural idiom of distress rather than a cultural syndrome and is not listed as such in DSM-5. In DSM-5, four cultural syndromes are listed and discussed in the "Glossary of Cultural Concepts of Distress" in the appendix: *dhat* syndrome, *khyâl cap*, *shenjing shuairuo*, and *taijin kyofusho*.

Dhat Syndrome

Dhat syndrome is a term that was coined in South Asia a little more than half a century ago to account for common clinical presentations of young male patients who attributed their various symptoms to semen loss. Despite the name, it is not a discrete syndrome but rather a cultural explanation of distress for patients who experience diverse symptoms such as anxiety, fatigue, weakness, weight loss, impotence, other somatic complaints, and depressive mood. The cardinal feature is anxiety and distress about the loss of *dhat* in the absence of any identifiable physiological dysfunction. *Dhat* is identified by patients as a white discharge noted on defecation or urination. Ideas about this substance are related to the concept of *dhatu* (semen) described in the Hindu system of medicine, *Ayurveda*, as one of seven essential bodily fluids whose balance is necessary in order to maintain health.

Although *dhat* syndrome was formulated as a cultural guide to local clinical practice, related ideas about the harmful effects of semen loss have been shown to be widespread in the general population (suggesting a cultural disposition for explaining health problems and symptoms). Although *dhat* syndrome is most commonly identified with young men from lower socioeconomic backgrounds, middle-age men may also be affected. Comparable concerns about white vaginal discharge (leukorrhea) have been associated with a variant of the concept for women.

Related conditions in other cultural contexts include *koro* in Southeast Asia, particularly Singapore, and *shen-k'uei* ("kidney deficiency") in China. Related conditions in DSM-5 are major depressive disorder, persistent depressive disorder (dysthymia), generalized anxiety disorder, somatic symptom disorder, illness anxiety disorder, erectile disorder, early (premature) ejaculation, other specified or unspecified sexual dysfunction, and academic problem.

Khyâl Cap

Khyâl attacks (*khyâl cap*), or "wind attacks," are a syndrome found among Cambodians in the United States and Cambodia. Common symptoms include those of panic attacks, such as dizziness, palpitations, shortness of breath, and cold extremities, as well as other symptoms of anxiety and autonomic arousal (e.g., tinnitus, neck soreness). *Khyâl* attacks include catastrophic cognitions centered on the concern that *khyâl* (a windlike substance) may rise in the body—along with blood—and cause a range of serious effects (e.g., compressing the lungs to cause shortness of breath and asphyxia; entering the cranium to cause tinnitus, dizziness, blurry vision, and a fatal syncope). *Khyâl* attacks may occur without warning but are frequently brought about by such triggers as worrisome thoughts, standing up (i.e., orthostasis), specific odors with negative associations, and agoraphobic-type cues such as going to crowded spaces or riding in a car. *Khyâl* attacks usually meet panic attack criteria and may shape the experience of other anxiety and trauma- and stressor-related disorders. *Khyâl* attacks may be associated with considerable disability.

Related conditions in other cultural contexts include *pen lom* (Laos), *srog rlung gi nad* (Tibet), *vata* (Sri Lanka), and *hwa-byung* (Korea). Related conditions in DSM-5 are panic attack, panic disorder, generalized anxiety disorder, agoraphobia, PTSD, and illness anxiety disorder.

Shenjing Shuairuo

Shenjing shuairuo ("weakness of the nervous system" in Mandarin Chinese) is a cultural syndrome that integrates conceptual categories of traditional Chinese medicine (TCM) with the Western diagnosis of neurasthenia. In the second, revised edition of the *Chinese Classification of Mental Disorders* (CCMD-2-R), *shenjing shuairuo* is defined as a syndrome composed of three out of five nonhierarchical symptom clusters: weakness (e.g., mental fatigue), emotions (e.g., feeling vexed), excitement (e.g., increased recollections), nervous pain (e.g., headache), and sleep (e.g., insomnia). *Fan nao* ("feeling vexed") is a form of irritability mixed with worry and distress over conflicting thoughts and unfulfilled desires.

The third edition of the CCMD retains *shenjing shuairuo* as a somatoform diagnosis of exclusion (Chang 2006). Salient precipitants of *shenjing shuairuo* include work- or family-related stressors, loss of face (*mianzi, lianzi*), and an acute sense of failure (e.g., in academic performance). *Shenjing shuairuo* is related to traditional concepts of weakness (*xu*) and health imbalances related to deficiencies of a vital essence (e.g., the depletion of *qi*) following overstraining or stagnation of *qi* due to excess worry. In the traditional interpretation, *shenjing shuairuo* results when bodily channels (*jing*) conveying vital forces (*shen*) become dysregulated as a result of various social and interpersonal stressors, such as the inability to change a chronically frustrating and distressing situation.

Related conditions in other cultural contexts include neurasthenia-spectrum idioms and syndromes in India (*ashaktapanna*), Japan (*shinkei suijaku*), and Nigeria (brain fag syndrome), among other settings. Other conditions, such as burnout syndrome and chronic fatigue syndrome, are also closely related. Related conditions in DSM-5 are major depressive disorder, persistent depressive disorder (dysthymia), generalized anxiety disorder, somatic symptom disorder, social anxiety disorder, specific phobia, and PTSD.

Taijin Kyofusho

Taijin kyofusho ("interpersonal fear disorder" in Japanese) is a cultural syndrome characterized by anxiety about and avoidance of interpersonal situations because of the thought, feeling, or conviction that one's appearance and actions in social interactions are inadequate or offensive to others (Iwata et al. 2011). Individuals with *taijin kyofusho* tend to focus on the impact of their symptoms and behaviors on others. Variants include major concerns about facial blushing (erythrophobia), having an offensive body odor (olfactory reference syndrome), inappropriate gaze (too much or too little eye contact), stiff or awkward facial expression or bodily movements (e.g., stiffening, trembling), or body deformity.

Taijin kyofusho is a broader construct than social anxiety disorder in DSM-5. In addition to performance anxiety, *taijin kyofusho* includes two culture-related forms: a sensitive type, with extreme social sensitivity and anxiety about interpersonal interactions, and an offensive type, in which the major concern is offending others. As a category, *taijin kyofusho* thus includes syndromes with features of body dysmorphic disorder as well as delusional disorder. The patient's concerns may have a delusional quality, and the patient may respond poorly to simple reassurance or counterexample.

The distinctive symptoms of *taijin kyofusho* occur in specific cultural contexts and, to some extent, with more severe social anxiety across cultures. Similar syndromes are found in Korea and other societies that place a strong emphasis on the self-conscious maintenance of appropriate social behavior in hierarchical interpersonal relationships. *Taijin kyofusho*–like symptoms have also been described in other cultural contexts, including the United States, Australia, and New Zealand.

A related condition in other cultural contexts is *taein kong po* in Korea. Related conditions in DSM-5 are social anxiety disorder, body dysmorphic disorder, delusional disorder, obsessive-compulsive disorder, and olfactory reference syndrome (a type of other specified obsessive-compulsive and related disorder). Olfactory reference syndrome is related specifically to the *jikoshu-kyofu* variant of *taijin kyofusho*, whose core symptom is the concern that the person emits an offensive body odor. This presentation is seen in various cultures outside Japan.

Treatment Modalities

Psychotic Disorders

Asian Americans underutilize mental health services (Abe-Kim et al. 2007), which may be related to a longer duration of untreated psychosis than is found in other ethnic groups (Ryder et al. 2000). Duration of untreated psychosis has been demonstrated to influence Positive and Negative Syndrome Scale (PANSS) scores and quality of life, making this an important factor in treatment outcomes (Kane et al. 2016). Help-seeking behavior in persons with mental illness can be seen as a several-step process. First, there is denial of the problem, which usually is followed by attempts by the family, extended family, and community to contain or conceal the problem. The first effort to obtain help outside the family usually is consultation with a traditional healer. Traditional healers are widely used in many cultures, both in conjunction with and in place of Western medicine (Ma 1999). It is important to understand some of the methods that may be employed by the traditional healer because they leave physical markings on the body that may be interpreted as signs of abuse. These methods, which may be used in the treatment of psychosis and other mental disorders to eliminate "bad wind" from the body, are coining, pinching, cupping, and moxibustion.

- *Coining* is the practice of using a coin or similar dull-edged object to superficially scratch a certain area on the body until the skin turns deep red to get the bad wind out of the body. The deeper the redness on the skin, the more bad wind has been released from the body. This method is applied mostly to the back or the back of the neck.
- In *pinching*, the traditional healer uses fingers to pinch the skin in sensitive areas until a contusion occurs, indicating that the bad wind has been removed or released.
- *Cupping* is a method of applying heated cups on the back, forehead, or abdomen to suck out the bad wind.
- *Moxibustion* involves burning incense or combustible herbs to cause superficial small burns on the torso, head, and neck to remove the bad wind (Wong et al. 1999).

Another major treatment consideration is the impact of ethnic and cultural factors on drug metabolism, treatment adherence, and treatment responsiveness. Some Asian Americans may require lower doses of antipsychotics because of differential expression of cytochrome P450 enzymes, especially 2D6 and 2C19. Similar considerations may be needed regarding appropriate dosage of medication in patients with treatment-resistant illness (Zhou et al. 2009). An important factor for consideration in pharmacological treatment adherence is English proficiency; diminished English proficiency has been shown to negatively impact adherence (Gilmer et al. 2009). Finally, when evaluating patients, it is imperative to obtain a complete history of recent use of all medications, including herbal remedies. Certain herbal medications, such as the Japanese *Swertia japonica* and *kamikihi-to*, have been shown to cause psychosis when combined with psychotropic medications (Faison and Armstrong 2013).

Mood Disorders

In treating mood disorders, as with other psychiatric conditions, it is important to inquire about alternative treatments, including use of traditional healers and herbal remedies. At the same time, open-mindedness toward alternative treatments is vital. A recent meta-analysis demonstrated *qigong* as an effective intervention to reduce depressive symptomatology (Liu et al. 2015).

Nonadherence remains a concern in treating Asians. Given the many barriers to engagement in psychiatric care, provision of care through primary care providers is incredibly important. One study demonstrated noninferiority of the collaborative care approach to Asian American mental health care outcomes, in comparison with Asian American mental health care delivered by a culturally sensitive community health center (Ratzliff et al. 2013). This allows for the possibility of using collaborative care approaches to improve access to appropriate mental health care for a broader population of Asian Americans.

In terms of psychopharmacological treatment, when prescribing selective serotonin reuptake inhibitors (SSRIs), the ones that have a more favorable side-effect profile should be considered first. Unfortunately, adherence cannot be monitored through blood levels. Patients who are accustomed to using herbal remedies to treat their symptoms will expect rapid relief and may consider the provider incompetent if they do not feel better quickly. Some providers may handle this situation by prescribing benzodiazepines to offer short-term symptom relief until SSRIs reach therapeutic levels. Patients also may stop taking their medications when they begin to feel better. Therefore, it is important to check in with the patient periodically to make certain he or she is still taking the medication. Explaining depression as a biochemical imbalance in the brain that requires continuous regulation with the medication can be helpful. As always, it is important to involve family in the treatment decision-making process.

Additional treatment options beyond pharmacotherapy remain important. Exercise has been shown to be effective among Korean Americans for depression and has been found to have a high degree of acceptability (Kim and Im 2015). Psychotherapy is another important tool, although varied attitudes toward engagement may decrease its utility (Abe-Kim et al. 2007). When offered, culturally adapted forms of psychotherapy have been found to be effective (Hwang et al. 2015).

Anxiety Disorders

Patients often will try to manage anxiety themselves with alternative or traditional treatment methods or may consult a practitioner who specializes in such treatments. However, some herbal tonics and formulations used by traditional healers can cause an increase in sympathetic activation. These patients may then go to a primary care practitioner, who may make referrals to psychiatry after the medical workup for the patient's complaints yields negative results. It is imperative that psychiatrists inquire about all forms of treatment that have been or are being used because the sympathetic activity may be misinterpreted as anxiety. Patients do seek treatment through a combination of these methods at the same time, so it is important to ask about the different methods used to cope with stress and anxiety. Patients often will expect rapid results and may discontinue treatment or seek treatment elsewhere if they feel that the treatment process is progressing too slowly. Education regarding expectations of how psychotropic medications work and typical time frames is thus very important.

Individual psychotherapy has been proven effective in the treatment of PTSD, but Asian patients with PSTD may have a difficult time with the Western psychotherapy concepts that emphasize individualism, mastery of nature, and freedom of choice. They also may have a harder time sharing the story of their trauma because of past experiences with betrayal and physical and psychological abuse. Culturally adapted forms of cognitive-behavioral therapy for PTSD have been developed, with positive outcomes, especially for Cambodian and Vietnamese refugees (Carter et al. 2012). Similar effectiveness has been found for specific phobias through the use of culturally adapted forms of exposure therapy (Pan et al. 2011), and in China, culturally adapted forms of cognitive-behavioral therapy for generalized anxiety disorder have been developed (Zhang et al. 2002). Additionally, Asian Americans struggling with PTSD report significant benefit from ethnicity-matched therapists, resulting in higher treatment retention and number of sessions, an important consideration when referring for treatment (Geiger 1994). Discrimination-focused group therapy and other PTSD treatments have been effective for those refugees who are veterans of wars and conflicts in Southeast Asia (Loo et al. 2007).

Substance Use Disorders

There are unique barriers to treatment engagement among many Asian American patients with substance use disorders. These barriers include attempts to minimize substance use disorders to save face and maintain harmony within the family, concerns about loss of confidentiality, and fear of deportation (Masson et al. 2013). Families often try to resolve the issue of substance use through confrontation of the individual by criticizing, threatening, or rejecting the person with the problem. Initially, immediate family members are brought in, and if they are unsuccessful, then members of the extended family or family friends may be included. An examination of Asian American attitudes toward treatment demonstrates a tendency among this population to use personal resources over professional or formal treatment programs in the context of substance use disorders (Lee et al. 2004). Only after these methods fail to bring about the desired response might the patient enter a treatment program.

Too often, given attitudes and barriers to treatment, Asian Americans engaging in treatment are motivated by involvement in the criminal justice system (Masson et al. 2013; Wu and Blazer 2015). The societal stigma associated with substance use often makes professional help a last resort. Notably, however, culturally competent service availability helps increase treatment utilization among Asian Americans, making this an important consideration when attempting to engage Asian Americans in substance use treatment (Yu et al. 2009). Despite a desire to save face and avoid shame, once engaged in treatment, Asian Americans are similar to other populations in treatment retention, completion, and outcome measures (Evans et al. 2012), although one study demonstrated better alcohol treatment outcomes for Asian Americans (Niv et al. 2007).

Dementia

Because of the strong family tradition of caregiving, Asian Americans tend to rely less on formal support and more on their families for dementia support. In one study among Korean Americans, family support and the importance of the family played a protective role in caregiver satisfaction (Lee and Choi 2013). In a recent survey, many (44%) Japanese American elders responded that they would prefer to receive end-of-life care at home, whereas only 12% preferred a nursing home (Fukui et al. 2013). In one study, Chinese Americans exhibited deficiencies in recognizing symptoms of dementia, which compromised help-seeking behavior (Diamond and Woo 2014). Among Korean Americans, a similar trend of low service utilization for cognitive impairment was also seen (Lee et al. 2014).

Given preconceived notions and culturally informed beliefs about dementia, psychoeducation plays an important role. An educational intervention aimed at Chinese Americans was found to increase positive affect among caregivers and to decrease distress associated with patient behaviors (Gallagher-Thompson et al. 2010). Because of the critically important role the family plays in dementia caregiving, involvement of family and caregivers is crucial, especially when discussing the diagnosis, treatment, and potential additional psychosocial supports that are available in the community.

CONCLUSION

Psychiatric illnesses faced by Asian Americans and Pacific Islanders in the United States are complicated by social and cultural barriers as well as issues with access to care, language barriers, and limits to the cultural knowledge of practitioners. Patients with certain conditions tend to present differently in this population, and they need to be evaluated with care and respect for culture and ethnicity. Patients who remain in touch with their native language and preserve strong ethnic ties tend to maintain lower rates of mental illness than are seen in most Americans, and this is a trend that could be used to protect against psychiatric complaints. More research is needed to provide clinicians with information that can help them evaluate the best ways to diagnose and treat mental health issues in these populations, particularly the elderly, and to best serve patients with cultural competency and concern for their unique needs.

KEY POINTS

- Asian Americans and Pacific Islanders are the fastest-growing population in the United States compared with any other racial group, and they encompass a diverse ethnic and cultural realm. There are some 43 different ethnic groups—28 Asian and 15 Pacific Islander—who speak at least 32 primary languages and a host of dialects, many of which are not spoken outside individuals' own communities.
- Asian families place a high value on the family and community. In most Asian families, there is a mutual interdependence among generations.
- Asian Americans endorse more stigma associated with mental illness generally, including major depression, than do non-Hispanic whites. As a group, older Asian Americans may focus on psychosocial issues as the cause of mental illness.

- Many elderly Asian Americans prefer to use alternative medical practices and self-care over professional treatment. When they do seek mental health treatment, a number of Asian Americans will use complementary or alternative medicine or visit a traditional healer before consulting a Western doctor.
- In Asia and among Asian refugees and immigrants, there are multiple functional somatic syndromes that are common anxiety presentations. Some of these could be considered as cultural concepts of distress, some as idioms of distress, and some as causal explanations.

Questions for Further Thought

1. According to the 2010 U.S. Census, what percentage of newly arrived immigrants have come from Asia?

    A. 16%.
    B. 26%.
    C. 36%.
    D. 46%.

2. When elderly immigrant Asian Americans seek treatment for a medical illness, which of the following are they most likely to see first?

    A. Community elder.
    B. Primary care physician.
    C. Hospital emergency department.
    D. Traditional healer.

3. Which of the following describes "semen loss?"

    A. *Dhat* syndrome.
    B. *Shenjing shuairuo.*
    C. *Hwa-byung.*
    D. *Khyâl cap.*

4. All of the following are traditional Asian healing methods used in the treatment of psychosis except

    A. Coining.
    B. Pinching.
    C. Cupping.
    D. Moxibustion.
    E. Sweat boxes.

5. Elderly immigrants from which of the following countries came primarily as political refugees?

    A. India.
    B. Vietnam.
    C. Singapore.
    D. South Korea.
    E. Japan.

6. Which of the following minority groups has the lowest incidence of dementia?

    A. Asian Americans.
    B. African Americans.
    C. Pacific Islanders.
    D. Alaska Natives.
    E. American Indians.

SUGGESTED READINGS AND WEBSITES

Evans E, Pierce J, Li L, et al: More alike than different: health needs, services utilization, and outcomes of Asian American and Pacific Islander (AAPI) populations treated for substance use disorders. J Ethn Subst Abuse 11(4):318–338, 2012 23216439

Jimenez DE, Bartels SJ, Cardenas V, et al: Cultural beliefs and mental health treatment preferences of ethnically diverse older adult consumers in primary care. Am J Geriatr Psychiatry 20(6):533–542, 2012 21992942

Kao RSK, Lam ML: Asian American elderly, in Working With Asian Americans: A Guide for Clinicians. Edited by Lee E. New York, Guilford, 1997, pp 208–223

Stanford Ethnogeriatrics curriculum, available at: https://geriatrics.stanford.edu

REFERENCES

Abe-Kim J, Takeuchi DT, Hong S, et al: Use of mental health-related services among immigrant and US-born Asian Americans: results from the National Latino and Asian American Study. Am J Public Health 97(1):91–98, 2007 17138905

Alarcón RD: Cultural inroads in DSM-5. World Psychiatry 13(3):310–313, 2014 25273305

Alzheimer's Association and Centers for Disease Control and Prevention: The Healthy Brain Initiative: The Public Health Road Map for State and National Partnerships, 2013–2018. Chicago, IL, Alzheimer's Association, 2013. Available at: https://alz.org/publichealth/downloads/2013-RoadMap.pdf. Accessed May 22, 2018.

American Psychiatric Association: Diagnostic and Statistical Manual of Mental Disorders, 4th Edition, Text Revision. Washington, DC, American Psychiatric Association, 2000

American Psychiatric Association: Diagnostic and Statistical Manual of Mental Disorders, 5th Edition. Arlington, VA, American Psychiatric Association, 2013

Aranda MP, Knight BG: The influence of ethnicity and culture on the caregiver stress and coping process: a sociocultural review and analysis. Gerontologist 37(3):342–354, 1997 9203758

Bartels SJ, Coakley E, Oxman TE, et al: Suicidal and death ideation in older primary care patients with depression, anxiety, and at-risk alcohol use. Am J Geriatr Psychiatry 10(4):417–427, 2002 12095901

Bignall WJR, Jacquez F, Vaughn LM: Attributions of mental illness: an ethnically diverse community perspective. Community Ment Health J 51(5):540–545, 2015 25536943

Breslau J, Aguilar-Gaxiola S, Borges G, et al: Risk for psychiatric disorder among immigrants and their US-born descendants: evidence from the National Comorbidity Survey Replication. J Nerv Ment Dis 195(3):189–195, 2007 17468677

Burnett-Zeigler I, Bohnert KM, Ilgen MA: Ethnic identity, acculturation and the prevalence of lifetime psychiatric disorders among black, Hispanic, and Asian adults in the U.S. J Psychiatr Res 47(1):56–63, 2013 23063326

Carter MM, Mitchell FE, Sbrocco T: Treating ethnic minority adults with anxiety disorders: current status and future recommendations. J Anxiety Disord 26(4):488–501, 2012 22417877

Chan SW: Family caregiving in dementia: the Asian perspective of a global problem. Dement Geriatr Cogn Disord 30(6):469–478, 2010 21252540

Chang D: Culture-bound syndromes: shenjing shuairuo, in Encyclopedia of Multicultural Psychology. Edited by Jackson Y. Thousand Oaks, CA, Sage, 2006, pp 144–144

Chen JA, Hung GC, Parkin S, et al: Illness beliefs of Chinese American immigrants with major depressive disorder in a primary care setting. Asian J Psychiatr 13:16–22, 2015 25563074

Chen YY, Wu KC, Yousuf S, et al: Suicide in Asia: opportunities and challenges. Epidemiol Rev 34(1):129–144, 2012 22158651

Cheng ST, Lam LC, Kwok T, et al: The social networks of Hong Kong Chinese family caregivers of Alzheimer's disease: correlates with positive gains and burden. Gerontologist 53(6):998–1008, 2013 23371974

Cheng TA: Sex difference in prevalence of minor psychiatric morbidity: a social epidemiological study in Taiwan. Acta Psychiatr Scand 80(4):395–407, 1989 2589095

Cho MJ, Lee JY, Kim BS, et al: Prevalence of the major mental disorders among the Korean elderly. J Korean Med Sci 26(1):1–10, 2011 21218022

Chopra D: What is Ayurveda? Carlsbad, CA, Chopra Center, 2017. Available at: www.chopra.com/articles/what-is-ayurveda#sm.000011b2s4yz96emwy16ubxy4c44q. Accessed December 8, 2017.

Diamond AG, Woo BK: Duration of residence and dementia literacy among Chinese Americans. Int J Soc Psychiatry 60(4):406–409, 2014 23828765

Duldulao AA, Takeuchi DT, Hong S: Correlates of suicidal behaviors among Asian Americans. Arch Suicide Res 13(3):277–290, 2009 19591001

Ekanayake S, Ahmad F, McKenzie K: Qualitative cross-sectional study of the perceived causes of depression in South Asian origin women in Toronto. BMJ Open 2(1):e000641, 2012 22337816

Evans E, Pierce J, Li L, et al: More alike than different: health needs, services utilization, and outcomes of Asian American and Pacific Islander (AAPI) populations treated for substance use disorders. J Ethn Subst Abuse 11(4):318–338, 2012 23216439

Faison WE, Armstrong D: Cultural aspects of psychosis in the elderly. J Geriatr Psychiatry Neurol 16(4):225–231, 2013 14653431

Feng Y, Wu Z, Zhou X, et al: Knowledge discovery in traditional Chinese medicine: state of the art and perspectives. Artif Intell Med 38(3):219–236, 2006 16930966

Fukui S, Fujita J, Yoshiuchi K: Associations between Japanese people's concern about famly caregiver burden and preference for end-of-life care location. J Palliat Care 29(1):22–28, 2013 23614167

Gallagher-Thompson D, Wang PC, Liu W, et al: Effectiveness of a psychoeducational skill training DVD program to reduce stress in Chinese American dementia caregivers: results of a preliminary study. Aging Ment Health 14(3):263–273, 2010 20425645

Gee K, Ishii M: Assessment and treatment of schizophrenia among Asian Americans, in Working With Asian Americans: A Guide for Clinicians. Edited by Lee E. New York, Guilford, 1997, pp 227–251

Geiger L: Ethnic match and client characteristics as predictors of treatment outcome for anxiety disorders. Diss Abstr Int 54:4387, 1994

Georg Hsu LK, Wan YM, Chang H, et al: Stigma of depression is more severe in Chinese Americans than Caucasian Americans. Psychiatry 71(3):210–218, 2008 18834272

Gilmer TP, Ojeda VD, Barrio C, et al: Adherence to antipsychotics among Latinos and Asians with schizophrenia and limited English proficiency. Psychiatr Serv 60(2):175–182, 2009 19176410

Helman CG: Culture, Health, and Illness: An Introduction for Health Professionals. London, Wright, 1990

Hinton DE, Park L, Hsia C, et al: Anxiety disorder presentations in Asian populations: a review. CNS Neurosci Ther 15(3):295–303, 2009 19691549

Hinton WL, Chen YC, Du N, et al: DSM-III-R disorders in Vietnamese refugees. Prevalence and correlates. J Nerv Ment Dis 181(2):113–122, 1993 8426168

Hwang WC, Myers HF, Chiu E, et al: Culturally adapted cognitive-behavioral therapy for Chinese Americans with depression: a randomized controlled trial. Psychiatr Serv 66(10):1035–1042, 2015 26129996

Iwata Y, Suzuki K, Takei N, et al: Jiko-shisen-kyofu (fear of one's own glance), but not taijin-kyofusho (fear of interpersonal relations), is an East Asian culture-related specific syndrome. Aust N Z J Psychiatry 45(2):148–152, 2011 21091156

Jackson JS, Abelson JM, Berglund PA, et al: Ethnicity, immigration, and cultural influences on the nature and distribution of mental disorders: an examination of major depression, in Conceptual Evolution of DSM-5. Edited by Regier D, Narrow W, Kuhl E, et al. Washington, DC, American Psychiatric Publishing, 2011, pp 267–285

Jenkins JH, Kleinman A, Good B: Cross-cultural studies of depression, in Psychosocial Aspects of Depression. Edited by Becker J, Kleinman A. Hillsdale, NJ, Erlbaum, 1990, pp 67–99

Jimenez DE, Alegría M, Chen CN, et al: Prevalence of psychiatric illnesses in older ethnic minority adults. J Am Geriatr Soc 58(2):256–264, 2010 20374401

Jimenez DE, Bartels SJ, Cardenas V, et al: Cultural beliefs and mental health treatment preferences of ethnically diverse older adult consumers in primary care. Am J Geriatr Psychiatry 20(6):533–542, 2012 21992942

Kane JM, Robinson DG, Schooler NR, et al: Comprehensive versus usual community care for first-episode psychosis: 2-year outcomes from the NIMH RAISE Early Treatment Program. Am J Psychiatry 173(4):362–372, 2016 26481174

Kao RSK, Lam ML: Asian American elderly, in Working With Asian Americans: A Guide for Clinicians. Edited by Lee E. New York, Guilford, 1997, pp 208–223

Karasz A: Cultural differences in conceptual models of depression. Soc Sci Med 60(7):1625–1635, 2005 15652693

Karasz A, Dempsey K, Fallek R: Cultural differences in the experience of everyday symptoms: a comparative study of South Asian and European American women. Cult Med Psychiatry 31(4):473–497, 2007 17985219

Kelley HH: The process of causal attribution. Am Psychol 28(2):107–128, 1973

Keshavan MS: Culture bound syndromes: disease entities or simply concepts of distress? Asian J Psychiatr 12:1–2, 2014 25440557

Kim E, Im EO: Korean-Americans' knowledge about depression and attitudes about treatment options. Issues Ment Health Nurs 36(6):455–463, 2015 26241572

Kim HS, Sherman DK, Ko D, et al: Pursuit of comfort and pursuit of harmony: culture, relationships, and social support seeking. Pers Soc Psychol Bull 32(12):1595–1607, 2006 17122173

Kirmayer LJ, Robbins JM: Patients who somatize in primary care: a longitudinal study of cognitive and social characteristics. Psychol Med 26(5):937–951, 1996 8878327

Kleinman AM: Depression, somatization and the "new cross-cultural psychiatry." Soc Sci Med 11(1):3–10, 1977 887955

Kleinman A: The cultural construction of illness experience and behavior, 2: a model of somatization of dysphoric affects and affective disorders, in Patients and Healer in the Context of Culture: An Exploration of the Borderland Between Anthropology, Medicine, and Psychiatry. Edited by Kleinman A. Berkeley, University of California Press, 1980, pp 146–178

Kleinman A, Eisenberg L, Good B: Culture, illness, and care: clinical lessons from anthropologic and cross-cultural research. Ann Intern Med 88(2):251–258, 1978 626456

Kulkarni RS, Shinde RL: Depression and its associated factors in older Indians. a study based on study of global aging and adult health (SAGE)-2007. J Aging Health 27(4):622–649, 2015 25370713

Kung WW, Lu PC: How symptom manifestations affect help seeking for mental health problems among Chinese Americans. J Nerv Ment Dis 196(1):46–54, 2008 18195641

Kuriyama S: The Divergence of Greek and Chinese Medicine. New York, Zone Books, 2002

La Fontaine J, Ahuja J, Bradbury NM, et al: Understanding dementia amongst people in minority ethnic and cultural groups. J Adv Nurs 60(6):605–614, 2007 18039247

Lai D, Chappell N: Use of traditional Chinese medicine by older Chinese immigrants in Canada. Fam Pract 24(1):56–64, 2007 17121747

Lee CK, Kwak YS, Yamamoto J, et al: Psychiatric epidemiology in Korea. Part II: urban and rural differences. J Nerv Ment Dis 178(4):247–252, 1990 2181056

Lee HB, Han HR, Huh BY, et al: Mental health service utilization among Korean elders in Korean churches: preliminary findings from the Memory and Aging Study of Koreans in Maryland (MASK-MD). Aging Ment Health 18(1):102–109, 2014 23889338

Lee MY, Law PF, Eo E: Perception of substance use problems in Asian American communities by Chinese, Indian, Korean, and Vietnamese populations. J Ethn Subst Abuse 2(3):1–29, 2004 29019292

Lee Y, Choi S: Korean American dementia caregivers' attitudes toward caregiving: the role of social network versus satisfaction with social support. J Appl Gerontol 32(4):422–442, 2013 25474683

Lin K-M, Cheung F: Mental health issues for Asian Americans. Psychiatr Serv 50(6):774–780, 1999 10375146

Lin SY: Beliefs about causes, symptoms, and stigma associated with severe mental illness among "highly acculturated" Chinese-American patients. Int J Soc Psychiatry 59(8):745–751, 2013 22885690

Lin TY: Psychiatry and Chinese culture. West J Med 139(6):862–867, 1983 6364576

Liu X: Psychiatry in traditional Chinese medicine. Br J Psychiatry 138:429–433, 1981 7025950

Liu X, Clark J, Siskind D, et al: A systematic review and meta-analysis of the effects of Qigong and Tai Chi for depressive symptoms. Complement Ther Med 23(4):516–534, 2015 26275645

Loo CM, Fairbank JA, Chemtob CM: Adverse race-related events as a risk factor for posttraumatic stress disorder in Asian American Vietnam veterans. J Nerv Ment Dis 193(7):455–463, 2005 15985840

Loo CM, Ueda SS, Morton RK: Group treatment for race-related stresses among minority Vietnam veterans. Transcult Psychiatry 44(1):115–135, 2007 17379613

Ma GX: Between two worlds: the use of traditional and Western health services by Chinese immigrants. J Community Health 24(6):421–437, 1999 10593423

Marshall GN, Schell TL, Elliott MN, et al: Mental health of Cambodian refugees 2 decades after resettlement in the United States. JAMA 294(5):571–579, 2005 16077051

Masson CL, Shopshire MS, Sen S, et al: Possible barriers to enrollment in substance abuse treatment among a diverse sample of Asian Americans and Pacific Islanders: opinions of treatment clients. J Subst Abuse Treat 44(3):309–315, 2013 22985677

Mayeda FR, Glymour MM, Quesenberry CP, et al: Inequalities in dementia incidence between six racial and ethnic groups over 14 years. Alzheimers Dement 12(3):216–224, 2016 26874595

Montenegro X: Are Asian Americans and Pacific Islanders financially secure? Washington, DC, AARP, March 2015. Available at: www.aarp.org/research/topics/economics/info-2015/asian-americans-pacific-islanders-financial-security.html. Accessed December 8, 2017.

Mui AC: Depression among elderly Chinese immigrants: an exploratory study. Soc Work 41(6):633–645, 1996 8900083

Najm W, Reinsch S, Hoehler F, et al: Use of complementary and alternative medicine among the ethnic elderly. Altern Ther Health Med 9(3):50–57, 2003 12776475

Niv N, Wong EC, Hser YI: Asian Americans in community-based substance abuse treatment: service needs, utilization, and outcomes. J Subst Abuse Treat 33(3):313–319, 2007 17376635

Pan D, Huey SJ Jr, Hernandez D: Culturally adapted versus standard exposure treatment for phobic Asian Americans: treatment efficacy, moderators, and predictors. Cultur Divers Ethnic Minor Psychol 17(1):11–22, 2011 21341893

Park S, Lee HB, Lee SY, et al: Trends in suicide methods and rates among older adults in South Korea: a comparison with Japan. Psychiatry Investig 13(2):184–189, 2016 27081378

Parker G, Cheah YC, Roy K: Do the Chinese somatize depression? A cross-cultural study. Soc Psychiatry Psychiatr Epidemiol 36(6):287–293, 2001 11583458

Pew Research Center: Family and personal values, in The Rise of Asian Americans. Washington, DC, Pew Research Center, June 19, 2012, pp 139–252. Available at: www.pewsocialtrends.org/2012/06/19/chapter-5-family-and-personal-values. Accessed December 8, 2017.

Ratzliff AD, Ni K, Chan YF, et al: A collaborative care approach to depression treatment for Asian Americans. Psychiatr Serv 64(5):487–490, 2013 23632577

Ryder AG, Bean G, Dion KL: Caregiver responses to symptoms of first-onset psychosis: a comparative study of Chinese- and Euro-Canadian families. Transcult Psychiatry 27:225–236, 2000

Seby K, Chaudhury S, Chakraborty R: Prevalence of psychiatric and physical morbidity in an urban geriatric population. Indian J Psychiatry 53(2):121–127, 2011 21772643

Sentell T, Unick GJ, Hyeong JA, et al: Illness severity and psychiatric hospitalization rates among Asian Americans and Pacific Islanders. Psychiatr Serv 64(11):1095–1102, 2013 23945849

Sue S, Chen J, Saad CS, et al: Asian American mental health: a call to action. Am Psychol 67(7):532–544, 2012 23046304

Tran C, Hinton L: Health and Health Care of Vietnamese American Older Adults. Stanford, CA, Stanford School of Medicine, 2010. Available at: http://geriatrics.stanford.edu/wp-content/uploads/downloads/ethnomed/vietnamese/downloads/vietnamese_american.pdf. Accessed December 11, 2017.

Uba L: Cultural barriers to health care for Southeast Asian refugees. Public Health Rep 107(5):544–548, 1992 1410235

U.S. Department of Health and Human Services: Mental Health: Culture, Race, and Ethnicity: A Report of the Surgeon General. Rockville, MD, Substance Abuse and Mental Health Services Administration, 2001

U.S. Department of Health and Human Services: Health, United States, 2011: With Special Feature on Socioeconomic Status and Health. Hyattsville, MD, National Center for Health Statistics, 2012. Available at: www.cdc.gov/nchs/data/hus/hus11.pdf. Accessed May 15, 2018

U.S. Department of Health and Human Services: National Plan to Address Alzheimer's Disease: 2017 Update. Washington, DC, Office of the Assistant Secretary for Planning and Evaluation. Available at: https://aspe.hhs.gov/system/files/pdf/257526/NatlPlan2017.pdf. Accessed: May 22, 2018.

Vaughn L, Jacquez F, Baker RC: Cultural health attributions, beliefs, and practices: effects on healthcare and medical education. The Open Medical Education Journal 2:64–74, 2009

Ventriglio A, Ayonrinde O, Bhugra D: Relevance of culture-bound syndromes in the 21st century. Psychiatry Clin Neurosci 70(1):3–6, 2016 26332813

Whaley AL: Ethnic and racial differences in perceptions of dangerousness of persons with mental illness. Psychiatr Serv 48(10):1328–1330, 1997 9323754

Wong HC, Wong JKT, Wong NYY: Signs of physical abuse or evidence of moxibustion, cupping or coining? CMAJ 160(6):785–786, 1999 10189420

World Health Organization: Disease and Injury Country Estimates. Geneva, Switzerland, World Health Organization, April 2011. Available at: www.who.int/healthinfo/global_burden_disease/estimates_country/en. Accessed May 11, 2018

Wu LT, Blazer DG: Substance use disorders and co-morbidities among Asian Americans and Native Hawaiians/Pacific Islanders. Psychol Med 45(3):481–494, 2015 25066115

Wu LT, Blazer D, Gersing KR et al: Comorbid substance use disorders with other Axis I and II mental disorders among treatment-seeking Asian Americans, Native Hawaiians/Pacific Islanders, and mixed-race people. J Psychiatr Res 47(12):1940–1948, 2013 24060266

Xu Y, Okuda M, Hser YI, et al: Twelve-month prevalence of psychiatric disorders and treatment-seeking among Asian Americans/Pacific Islanders in the United States: results from the National Epidemiological Survey on Alcohol and Related Conditions. J Psychiatr Res 45(7):910–918, 2011 21238989

Yang LH, WonPat-Borja AJ: Psychopathology among Asian Americans, in Handbook of Asian American Psychology, 2nd Edition. Edited by Leong FTL, Ebreo A, Kinoshita L, et al. Thousand Oaks, CA, Sage, 2006, pp 379–405

Yeung A, Kam R: Illness beliefs of depressed Asian Americans in primary care, in Perspectives in Cross-Cultural Psychiatry. Edited by Georgiopoulos AM, Rosenbaum JF. Philadelphia, PA, Lippincott Williams & Wilkins, 2005, pp 21–36

Yeung A, Chang D, Gresham RL Jr, et al: Illness beliefs of depressed Chinese American patients in primary care. J Nerv Ment Dis 192(4):324–327, 2004 15060408

Yu J, Clark LP, Chandra L, et al: Reducing cultural barriers to substance abuse treatment among Asian Americans: a case study in New York City. J Subst Abuse Treat 37(4):398–406, 2009 19553065

Zhang J, Fang L, Wu YW, et al: Depression, anxiety, and suicidal ideation among Chinese Americans: a study of immigration-related factors. J Nerv Ment Dis 201(1):17–22, 2013 23274290

Zhang Y, Young D, Lee S, et al: Chinese Taoist cognitive psychotherapy in the treatment of generalized anxiety disorder in contemporary China. Transcult Psychiatry 39(1):115–129, 2002

Zhong BL, Chiu HF, Conwell Y: Rates and characteristics of elderly suicide in China, 2013–14. J Affect Disord 206:273–279, 2016 27639861

Zhou SF, Liu JP, Chowbay B: Polymorphism of human cytochrome P450 enzymes and its clinical impact. Drug Metab Rev 41(2):89–295, 2009 19514967

CHAPTER 5

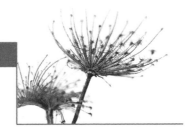

Culturally Competent Care for Geriatric Indigenous Peoples

AMERICAN INDIANS, ALASKA NATIVES, FIRST NATIONS, AND NATIVE HAWAIIANS

Mary Hasbah Roessel, M.D.

Linda Nahulu, M.D.

Mira Zein, M.D., M.P.H.

Learning Objectives

Gain an understanding and appreciate the diversity and complexity of Indigenous peoples of North America in order to identify cultural factors of Indigenous elderly when establishing rapport in clinical settings.

Acquire knowledge of the historical trauma that has occurred and recognize how it has impacted the Indigenous elderly in order to create a safe and healing environment.

Become familiar with traditional Indigenous healing practices that are integrated into Indigenous elderly lifestyles and help support this strength within these Indigenous elderly.

The Indigenous peoples of North America, or Turtle Island as it is called by the North American Indigenous nations, had more than 15 million original inhabitants in the United States alone and spoke more than 300 distinct languages. Now there are approximately 3 million Indigenous peoples in the United States, belonging to more than 500 federally recognized nations. It is important to note that Indigenous peoples now live mostly in urban centers rather than on reservations or trust lands. Each nation has its own language and cultural traditions, and, as a group, these nations are very diverse. There are many terms of reference for the Indigenous nations, including American Indian (AI), Alaska Native (AN), Native American, Indigenous, Native Hawaiian, First Nations, and Aboriginal (Dunbar-Ortiz 2014). Indigenous peoples prefer to be called by their individual nation or village name.

History

We Indigenous peoples have principles of being stewards of the land we inhabit and recognize a shared responsibility for the land and its resources. The Haida Gwaii First Nations in Canada have a guiding value that "the land does not belong to us," asserting that "we belong to the land."

Having an accurate history of the colonization of the Americas is necessary to understand the unique place in history of Indigenous peoples. Genocidal practices through massacres, forced relocations, and rupture of Native American (including First Nations, AN, and Native Hawaiian) families and cultures was pervasive in the settlement of North America. The Indigenous inhabitants of Turtle Island were imprisoned for practicing their ceremonies and cultural events. For example, in Canada, the Potlatch, a time of sharing food and goods, was outlawed. Throughout Turtle Island from the 1800s until the 1970s, children were taken away from their families and sent to residential or boarding schools, where they were punished for speaking their own languages and practicing their culture.

There were several significant periods in the history of North America that represent the genocidal practices of the Canadian and United States governments. Many Indigenous people today have direct family connections to the trauma from forced relocations and extermination policies. Examples include the Navajo (Diné) Long Walk (Hwéeldi) of 1864, a 300-mile forced march of 8,000 Navajo women, children, and men to a military internment camp in southern New Mexico, and the Cherokee Trail of Tears in 1838, a forced march of Cherokee women and children from Cherokee homelands in what is now Georgia and Alabama to Oklahoma (Dunbar-Ortiz 2014).

Subsequently, beginning with the U.S. policy of the General Allotment Act of 1887 and continuing until the 1960s, forced assimilation and land appropriations led to the termination of more than 100 Indigenous nations and the seizure and settlement of Indigenous lands by non- Indigenous peoples (Dunbar-Ortiz 2014). In the United States, the government created federally recognized reservations, and in Canada such reservations were called Reserves. Many of these reservations and Reserves were not on Indigenous sacred homelands. This historical trauma of the Indigenous peoples of Turtle Island has resulted in inter-generational trauma (Brave Heart and DeBruyn 1998). Many generations of Indigenous children and families have been traumatized from the past forced removal of their grandparents and parents and from being placed in boarding schools or residential schools. Indigenous families have been overwhelmingly impacted by this rupture that prevented their spiritual practices, culture, sacred lands, and family values from being passed on through each generation. The high rates of substance use disorders, posttraumatic stress disorder, suicide, and attachment disorders in many Indigenous peoples have been linked directly to the intergenerational historical trauma forced on them (Heart et al. 2011).

Indigenous people are resilient and are in the process of healing through reconciliation, reclaiming sacred lands and spiritual practices, and language. Indigenous peoples have a reciprocal relationship to Turtle Island and are at the forefront of being protectors of the water and lands that are being impacted by climate change. Indigenous peoples have, as a core value, reverence for the elders of their community and families. Indigenous elders are looked to for the sacred teachings and have a role in family or community gatherings to start off the events with prayer. The elders are the carriers of the traditional knowledge within the Indigenous communities and often are spiritual leaders or Hatathli (medicine people) in the community. These familial or clan (Ké) roles and other roles in the Indigenous communities ensure sustainability and reciprocity for meaningful and long-standing tribal relationships. This is how the spiritual practices and traditions are carried on through each generation.

Cultural awareness of the significance of the roles of elders in Indigenous communities is just one factor in being culturally competent when providing psychiatric services to the Indigenous population. Mistrust of the health care system by Indigenous people has been a barrier for receiving services, so it is imperative for psychiatric providers to become knowledgeable about the Indigenous people they serve to avoid stereotyping and racism. When an Indigenous person makes the decision to pursue Western medical psychiatric services, that can be an intimidating process, and having a welcoming provider who is culturally sensitive will reduce that intimidation. "Culturally competent care builds trust, increasing the likelihood that Aboriginal people will go for care and stay in their treatment" (Health Council of Canada 2012, p. 4).

BELIEFS REGARDING ILLNESS, WELLNESS, AND MENTAL ILLNESS

Culture-Bound Syndromes (Cultural Concepts of Distress)

Many cultures conceptualize illness in ways that differ from those of Western medicine and psychiatry, and Indigenous people throughout the world still describe illness in these ways. In DSM-5, the terminology *culture-bound syndromes* was updated to *cultural concepts of distress* (American Psychiatric Association 2013). This updated description is an attempt to update these concepts and more accurately characterize the cultural influences on the expression and experience of mental disorders that occur in a person.

Ghost sickness is a preoccupation with death and the deceased. It is frequently described in Indigenous peoples, especially the Navajo (Diné). The symptoms are dizziness, bad dreams, fear, anxiety, fainting, and a sense of suffocation (Faison and Armstrong 2003). The Navajo believe ghost sickness is caused by exposure to death or by being bewitched by supernatural, evil powers. There are specific Navajo ceremonies that can cure it.

Arctic hysteria, or *pibloktoq,* is a dissociative episode in which a patient experiences prolonged extreme excitement, sometimes followed by seizures and coma. A prodrome can be irritability, and during the episode, the patient can exhibit dangerous, irrational behavior. Researchers have hypothesized that it is caused by vitamin A toxicity. Polar bear, seal, and walrus meat, which is a large part of the diet of Inuit, Inupiat, and Aleut people, has high levels of vitamin A. There also is a hypothesis that *pibloktoq* may be caused by malnutrition or vitamin D or calcium deficiency (Higgs 2011).

Treatment Modalities

Culturally appropriate treatment depends on an individual's tribal affiliation, level of traditional beliefs, and acculturation to the Western biomedical health care system. Elderly AIs, ANs, and other Indigenous peoples have had differing exposure to Western allopathic medicine through Indian Health Service (IHS) units or care in urban clinics or military settings. However, traditional healing practices and ceremonies are an important part of AI/AN and Indigenous culture, and available research points to increased utilization of integrated treatment modalities that incorporate traditional approaches to health and Western medicine (American Psychiatric Association Office of Minority and National Affairs 2010; Substance Abuse and Mental Health Services Administration et al. 2016). Historical trauma also should be considered in the treatment of mental health issues in the Native American elderly because intergenerational trauma has a significant impact on mental health and can often lead to distrust of Western modalities of treatment (American Psychiatric Association Office of Minority and National Affairs 2010; Substance Abuse and Mental Health Services Administration et al. 2016; U.S. Department of Health and Human Services 2017).

Traditional healing systems function on the basis of the traditional cultural outlook that mind, body, and spirit are interwoven with family, community, and land. Contrary to the Western biomedical approach, traditional healing does not try to isolate one part of the person and heal it but instead looks at the whole person in connection with social and ecological factors. Traditional treatments include ritual; ceremony; drumming; beading (sewing beaded objects); specific songs; fasting; sweating; herbal and/or animal medicines; and avoidance or inclusion of specific indigenous foods, natural elements, or situations, usually prescribed by a medicine person, spiritual advisor, or diagnostician, depending on tribal tradition and availability (American Psychiatric Association Office of Minority and National Affairs 2010; U.S. Department of Health and Human Services 2017).

Consideration of these traditional healing systems is incredibly important in the treatment of all AIs/ANs and other Indigenous peoples (including the elderly) because help seeking from traditional healers is common. Indigenous men and women who meet criteria for depression, anxiety, or substance use are significantly more likely to seek help from traditional spiritual healers than from other sources. In one study, 34%–49% of AIs/ANs diagnosed with behavioral disorders used traditional healers, and 16%–32% who were getting treatment from a Western medical source for a behavioral disorder had also seen a traditional healer (Beals et al. 2005; Walls et al. 2006).

In qualitative studies conducted by Dickerson et al. (2012), the Los Angeles County Department of Mental Health, and the UC Davis Center for Reducing Health Disparities, local AI/AN populations highlighted their belief that 1) cultural traditions and values were extremely important for physical, emotional, and spiritual health; 2) disconnection with their culture and heritage contributed to the fragmentation of their communities and to increased rates of substance use, depression, and suicide; and 3) tradition-based healing practices have the potential to help address the mental health care needs of their populations (Dickerson et al. 2012; UC Davis Center for Reducing Health Disparities 2009).

There have been numerous grassroots interventions established in AI/AN centers as well as urban centers across the country. A literature review by the Urban Indian Health Institute (2012) analyzed the scientific literature and systematically assessed various integrated treatment programs implemented by different tribes across the United States to treat depression and other common mental health concerns. The researchers found that key elements to successfully treating Native populations included the following:

- Focus on family and community, not just the individual, in prevention and treatment
- Incorporate traditional knowledge and practices
- Focus on active skills building (e.g., communication, coping, conflict management)
- Integrate and link treatment with prevention, particularly in places not associated with mental illness
- Expand cultural competency of both providers and health care systems
- Develop flexible provider-patient relationships with adaptive treatment approaches
- Implement environmental and structural changes to affect surrounding conditions
- Develop policies, systems, and adequate funding to improve health care and economic opportunities for AI/AN people

EXAMPLES OF INTEGRATED TREATMENT MODALITIES

DARTNA Protocol

Drum-Assisted Recovery Therapy for Native Americans (DARTNA) is a behavior therapy utilizing drumming therapy that was developed to treat AIs/ANs with substance use disorders (Dickerson et al. 2012). The concept behind use of drumming is that it is a common element used in sacred ceremonies as well as healing ceremonies in different tribal traditions, and it also has been shown to have potentially positive benefits in general substance use treatment and behavior change. DARTNA incorporates drumming, talking circles, and the White Bison conceptual framework. White Bison integrates the 12 steps of Alcoholics Anonymous and Narcotics Anonymous with the holistic health framework of the Medicine Wheel to emphasis AI values as part of sobriety. In an open pretest, 10 AIs with a history of substance use disorders participated in the DARTNA protocol and reported that they maintained sobriety or reduced their use of alcohol or other substances (Dickerson et al. 2014). Additionally, statistically significant improvements were found in indicators of medical, psychiatric, spiritual, and overall functional statuses.

Wind River Reservation–Wyoming State Hospital Collaboration

Wyoming State Hospital, an inpatient psychiatric hospital, operates in collaboration with members of the nearby Wind River Reservation and AI patients to develop services more acceptable to AIs and to incorporate traditional activities. On the basis of this collaboration, the tribe and hospital built a sweat lodge in a private area of the hospital grounds. Since its construction, there have been four to five sweat lodge ceremonies per year led by tribal elders or reservation officials. Use of the sweat lodge in combination with a dual-diagnosis program for persons with substance abuse and mental health issues has resulted in 1) improved utilization of the state hospital through increased referrals from the Reservation and IHS and increased AI inpatient admissions, 2) decreased length of stay for AI patients, 3) increased patient and tribal satisfaction, 3) improved health care outcomes for AI patients, and 4) improved collaboration between the hospital, tribe, and IHS (Tolman and Reedy 1998).

Holistic System of Care

The Native American Health Center in the San Francisco Bay Area developed Holistic System of Care (HSOC), a community-focused intervention aimed at providing behavioral, medical, and preventive services for urban AIs/ANs with comorbid conditions, including alcohol or substance abuse, mental health issues, and HIV/AIDS (Nebelkopf and Penagos 2005). The HSOC combines evidence-based and best practices (e.g., the Gathering of Native Americans curriculum for community healing and substance abuse prevention and recovery, motivational interviewing, and Positive Indian Parenting) with traditional AI/AN cultural practices, including smudging (an herbal cloud used in purification or healing ceremonies), traditional healers, powwows, sweat lodge ceremonies, seasonal ceremonies, and talking circles. Services all integrate a focus on family, community, Native culture, and recognizing historical trauma. Additionally, the HSOC includes practical support to address environmental factors influencing mental health and substance abuse, including life skills education, employment and housing services, positive peer role modeling, and community service.

Six-month follow-up evaluation results of the HSOC showed statistically significant decreases in serious depression, serious anxiety or tension, and attempted suicide and increased use of prescription psychological medication (Wright et al. 2011). In another study, treatment through the HSOC demonstrated statistically significant changes, including decreases in substance use; increases in employment; increases in school or training program enrollments; and decreases in serious depression, serious anxiety, trouble controlling violence, and suicide attempts (Nebelkopf and Wright 2011).

ASSESSMENT OF AND INITIATING TREATMENT FOR OLDER AMERICAN INDIAN/ALASKA NATIVES

Elder vs. Elderly

The term *elder* in the Indian community denotes a position of leadership based on experience, spirituality, and community service rather than age. There are elders in their 40s and 50s, and many Indian grandparents are in their late 30s. Therefore, elders are often distinguished from older AIs. Most IHS agencies consider the elderly to be persons 55 years and older. However, many tribes consider elderly to mean 50 years and older, and Medicare and Social Security consider 65 years to be the age of eligibility for benefits (Hendrix 2002).

Appropriate Ways to Show Respect and Establish Rapport

It is important to obtain a detailed history in a respectful manner in order to understand as much of the tribal and cohort influence on the individual as possible and to acknowledge the respect attributed to the wisdom of older individuals in AI/AN communities (Wright et al. 2011). Staff members providing care should be educated on tribally specific traditional narratives, beliefs, and practices and should be culturally competent (Brave Heart and DeBruyn 1998). Communication guidelines for assessment and treatment of AI/AN elderly can be found in Hendrix (2002).

Listening is valued over talking by most older AIs/ANs; calmness and humility are valued over speed and self-assertion or directedness. Many AI/AN elderly experience the "invisible elder" syndrome: Once revered in and the center of tribal life, seniors are now forgotten and, at times, abandoned by their children. To address this important concern, one should ask for the elder's help in understanding the current situation and in planning the components of further care.

Culturally Appropriate Verbal and Nonverbal Communication

Questions should be adapted to age and acculturation level. It is important for the health care provider to slow down when communicating with an Indian elder, especially during initial encounters and when explanations of treatments, medications, and health care decisions are being given. Questions should be carefully framed to convey the message of caring and should not indicate idle curiosity about the elder's culture or cultural practices.

Conversational Pace

AI languages have some of the longest pause times compared with other languages, especially English. Elders frequently complain that English speakers "talk too fast." Silence is valued, and long periods of silence between speakers are common. Interruption of the person who is speaking is considered extremely rude, especially if that person is an elder.

Nonverbal Communication

Health care providers should be aware of the following nonverbal characteristics:

- The usual comfort zone for physical distance is several feet.
- Eye contact is not direct or is only briefly direct; gaze may be directed over the shoulder.
- Emotional expressiveness may be controlled, except for humor.
- Body movements tend to be minimal.
- Touch is not usually acceptable, except for a handshake.

A Note on Prescribing Medication

Sharing of medicines (Indigenous and biomedical) is common within groups and extended families. The AI/AN patient may stop taking pharmaceuticals when he or she feels better, keeping extra medications to use later if the problem recurs. Many AI/AN patients will take Indigenous medicines prepared by a traditional healer concurrently with Western pharmaceutical medicines. Cost of medications can be a major factor in their use by AI/AN elderly, especially in urban or rural areas where IHS benefits are not available (Higgs 2011; Wright et al. 2011).

Next Steps: Research, Education, and Access to Care

Numerous barriers still remain that limit access to health care for AIs/ANs, including economic and financial barriers, limited data and research on health care for AIs/ANs, limited access to mental health professionals. and a lack of appropriate intervention strategies. The National Tribal Behavioral Health Agenda (Substance Abuse and Mental Health Services Administration et al. 2016) calls for increased funding for programs as well as funding for research to further elucidate the benefits of traditional interventions (Brave Heart and DeBruyn 1998). Supporting current programs, providing education to providers around culturally competent care, and advocating for policies that promote health equity are important next steps in improving mental health treatment for AI peoples.

KEY POINTS

- Indigenous peoples of North America are a diverse group, and approaching patients from their own cultural orientation and identity will assist in establishing rapport.
- Awareness of the colonization and historical trauma that have impacted many generations of Indigenous people will help providers engage in sensitive and nonjudgmental treatment with Indigenous patients.
- Being open to the continuing practice of traditional healing among Indigenous peoples is necessary for cultural awareness with Indigenous patients.

QUESTIONS FOR FURTHER THOUGHT

1. Indigenous peoples after colonization had their culture and lands reduced as well as which of the following?

   A. Their languages were reduced from more than 300 distinct languages.
   B. They lost cultural practices and were banned from practicing their ceremonies for hundreds of years.
   C. Tribal groups were reduced from more than 15 million people to 3 million people.
   D. All of the above.

2. Intergenerational trauma in Indigenous peoples has been linked to various psychiatric issues, including which of the following?

   A. Lower rates of PTSD.
   B. Low IQ scores.
   C. High rates of attachment disorders.
   D. High rates of eating disorders.

3. True or False: Culture-bound syndromes (cultural concepts of distress in DSM-5) characterize the cultural influences on the expression and experience of mental disorders that can occur in a person.

4. Which cultural treatment modality has been effective with Indigenous elderly?

   A. Seeking out culturally appropriate healing ceremonies.
   B. Use of talking circles.
   C. Integrating Indigenous art and aesthetics into the Western medical clinical setting.
   D. A and C.
   E. All of the above.

SUGGESTED READINGS AND WEBSITES

Doka K: Disenfranchised grief, in Living With Grief: Loss in Later Life. Edited by Doka KJ. Washington, DC, Hospice Foundation of America, 2002, pp 159–168

Dunbar-Ortiz R: An Indigenous Peoples' History of the United States. Boston, MA, Beacon, 2014

King T: The Inconvenient Indian: A Curious Account of Native People in North America. Toronto, ON, Canada, Anchor Canada, 2013

National Museum of the American Indian: http://nmai.si.edu

REFERENCES

American Psychiatric Association: Diagnostic and Statistical Manual of Mental Disorders, 5th Edition. Arlington, VA, American Psychiatric Association, 2013

American Psychiatric Association Office of Minority and National Affairs: Mental Health Disparities: American Indians and Alaska Natives (APA Fact Sheet). Arlington, VA, American Psychiatric Association, 2010. Available at: www.integration.samhsa.gov/workforce/mental_health_disparities_american_indian_and_alaskan_natives.pdf. Accessed December 20, 2017.

Beals J, Manson SM, Whitesell NR, et al: Prevalence of DSM-IV disorders and attendant help-seeking in 2 American Indian reservation populations. Arch Gen Psychiatry 62(1):99–108, 2005 15630077

Brave Heart MYH, DeBruyn IM: The American Indian Holocaust: healing historical unresolved grief. Am Indian Alsk Native Ment Health Res 8(2):56–78, 1998 9842066

Dickerson D, Robichaud F, Teruya C, et al: Utilizing drumming for American Indians/Alaska Natives with substance use disorders: a focus group study. Am J Drug Alcohol Abuse 38(5):505–510, 2012 22931086

Dickerson DL, Venner KL, Duran B, et al: Drum-Assisted Recovery Therapy for Native Americans (DARTNA): results from a pretest and focus groups. Am Indian Alsk Native Ment Health Res 21(1):35–58, 2014 24788920

Dunbar-Ortiz R: An Indigenous Peoples' History of the United States. Boston, MA, Beacon, 2014

Faison WE, Armstrong D: Cultural aspects of psychosis in the elderly. J Geriatr Psychiatry Neurol 16(4):225–231, 2003 14653431

Health Council of Canada: Empathy, Dignity, and Respect: Creating Cultural Safety for Aboriginal People in Urban Health Care. Toronto, ON, Canada, Health Council of Canada, December 2012. Available at: http://learning-circle.ubc.ca/files/2014/05/Empathy-dignity-and-respect-Creating-cultural-safety-for-Aboriginal-people-in-urban-health-care.pdf. Accessed December 20, 2017.

Heart MY, Chase J, Elkins J, et al: Historical trauma among Indigenous Peoples of the Americas: concepts, research, and clinical considerations. J Psychoactive Drugs 43(4):282–290, 2011 22400458

Hendrix LR: Health and health care of American Indian and Alaska Native elders. Ethnogeriatric Curriculum Module. Stanford, CA, Stanford Geriatric Education Center, 2002. Available at: http://web.stanford.edu/group/ethnoger/americanindian.html. Accessed December 22, 2017.

Higgs RD: Pibloktoq: A study of cultural-bound syndrome in the circumpolar region. Macalester Review 1:1–9, 2011

Nebelkopf E, Penagos M: Holistic Native network: integrated HIV/AIDS, substance abuse, and mental health services for Native Americans in San Francisco. J Psychoactive Drugs 37(3):257–264, 2005 16295008

Nebelkopf E, Wright S: Holistic System of Care: a ten-year perspective. J Psychoactive Drugs 43(4):302–308, 2011 22400461

Substance Abuse and Mental Health Services Administration, Tribal Technical Advisory Committee, Indian Health Services, National Indian Health Board: The National Tribal Behavioral Health Agenda. Washington, DC, Substance Abuse and Mental Health Services Administration, December 2016. Available at: http://store.samhsa.gov/shin/content//PEP16-NTBH-AGENDA/PEP16-NTBH-AGENDA.pdf. Accessed December 20, 2017.

Tolman A, Reedy R: Implementation of a culture-specific intervention for a Native American community. J Clin Psychol Med Settings 5(3):381–392, 1998

UC Davis Center for Reducing Health Disparities: Building Partnerships: Conversations With Native Americans About Mental Health Needs and Community Strengths. Sacramento, CA, UC Davis Center for Reducing Health Disparities, March 2009. Available at: www.dhcs.ca.gov/services/MH/Documents/BP_Native_American.pdf. Accessed December 21, 2017.

Urban Indian Health Institute: Addressing Depression Among American Indians and Alaska Natives: A Literature Review. Seattle Indian Health Board, August 2012. Available at: www.uihi.org/wp-content/uploads/2012/08/Depression-Environmental-Scan_All-Sections_2012-08-21_ES_FINAL.pdf. Accessed December 21, 2017.

U.S. Department of Health and Human Services: Health Conditions and Behaviors of Native Hawaiian and Pacific Islander Persons in the United States, 2014. Washington, DC, U.S. Department of Health and Human Services, July 2017. Available at: www.cdc.gov/nchs/data/series/sr_03/sr03_040.pdf. Accessed May 10, 2018.

Walls ML, Johnson KD, Whitbeck LB, et al: Mental health and substance abuse services preferences among American Indian people of the northern Midwest. Community Ment Health J 42(6):521–535, 2006 17143732

Wright S, Nebelkopf E, King J, et al: Holistic system of care: evidence of effectiveness. Subst Use Misuse 46(11):1420–1430, 2011 21810076

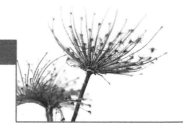

CHAPTER 6

African American Older Adults

Rita Hargrave, M.D.

Learning Objectives

Increase awareness of the impact of demographics, structural limitations of the U.S. health care system, and unique cultural values and health beliefs on psychiatric disorders among African American older adults.

Describe prevalence of and protective and risk factors for psychiatric disorders among African American older adults.

Describe the evidence-based pharmacological and behavioral interventions that are efficacious for mental disorders of African American older adults and describe areas for further research.

In 2013, 21.2% of persons age 65 and older were members of racial or ethnic minority populations; 8.6% were African Americans (West et al. 2014). The number of African American older adults is predicted to grow from 4 million in 2014 to 12 million by 2060 (Administration for Community Living 2017). This epidemiological trend underscores the importance of elucidating the psychiatric diagnostic and treatment issues of this population. In this chapter, I summarize the current knowledge of the mental health issues of African American older adults and provide suggestions for future research.

DEMOGRAPHICS, VALUES, AND UNIQUE FEATURES OF THE POPULATION

Geographic Distribution

From 1910 to 1970, an estimated 6 million African Americans left the segregation and discrimination of the South and settled in manufacturing centers in the Northeast and Midwest. Chicago, Detroit, New York City, and Philadelphia emerged as magnets for the social movement that became known as the Great Migration. In the 1940s, this social movement spread to even more cities across the Northeast, Midwest, and West (U.S. Census Bureau 2012).

Poverty

In 2014, the poverty rate for African Americans was 26.2%, compared with 14.8% nationally (DeNavas-Walt and Proctor 2015). African American retirees have significantly less wealth and lower incomes than white retirees. Eighty-three percent of African American seniors lack the retirement assets they need to last the remainder of their lifetimes (Meschede et al. 2011). Additionally, more than two-thirds of African Americans are liquid asset poor, meaning that their combined assets alone are not enough to make ends meet (Tippett 2014).

Education

In 1970, more than 50% of whites were high school graduates, but only 30% of African Americans had completed high school (U.S. Census Bureau 1999, Figure 4.1, p. 160). By 2016, 88.3% of whites had completed high school, compared with 76.4% of African Americans (National Center for Education Statistics 2017).

Support Networks

African American older adults often receive financial, instrumental, and emotional support from a broad social network consisting of family members and fictive kin (Becker et al. 2003). Fictive kin are individuals who are unrelated by either blood or marriage but uphold traditional family emotional and social obligations (Chatters et al. 1994). Fictive kin may include peer group members, godparents, or church members (Chatters et al. 1994; Taylor et al. 2005).

Health Beliefs Regarding Physical and Mental Illness

African American health beliefs and behaviors are deeply rooted in West African cultural traditions and the corrosive American slave experience. Patterns of health care utilization are closely related to social histories, health beliefs, cultural values, and attitudes (Hines-Martin et al. 2004; Ravenell et al. 2006). These influences may contribute to ethnic differences in health status and outcomes and health-seeking behaviors for mental health treatment (Dunlop et al. 2002; Snowden 2001). Knowledge of these core principles is necessary in order to design and target interventions to promote health-seeking behaviors and decrease health care disparities for African American older adults.

West African health traditions reflect a holistic ideology in which good health is the result of a harmonious relationship with nature and man (Spector 2013; Watson 1984). Disease is classified under three headings:1) natural (i.e., physical causes) (Simpson 1980; Tallant 1946), 2) occult (i.e., supernatural forces), or 3) spiritual ("due to willful violation of sacred beliefs" or sin (Mitchell 1978). According to West African traditions, natural illnesses are treated with homeopathic remedies. Among enslaved Africans, mistrust of and limited access to medical care, coupled with enduring West African folk traditions, promoted the widescale practice of folk medicine on the plantations (Covey 2007). Remnants of folk medicine have been passed down for generations and remain active in modern health care practices among African Americans.

The legacy of slavery exerts other powerful effects on African Americans' attitudes toward formalized health care. Slaves often were denied access to physicians until they were seriously ill (Washington 2007). Some researchers have suggested that slavery's marginal health service delivery may explain twenty-first-century elderly African Americans' pattern of accessing medical care at later stages of disease. Many of these elders seek care only when their illness is so far advanced that they cannot manage their activities of daily living (Martin et al. 2010). In addition, enslaved African Americans were subjected to harsh, abusive practices from medical providers. White physicians prescribed harsh treatments with hazardous agents and regularly condoned whippings to coerce ill slaves, accused of feigning their maladies, into working. Slaves frequently served as unwilling subjects in medical research, including surgical procedures conducted without use of anesthesia (Gamble 1997).

The U.S. Public Health Service's Tuskegee Study of Untreated Syphilis in the Negro Male (Rivers et al. 1953) was one infamous example of medical exploitation. From 1932 to 1972, 600 African Americans, lured by the promise of free health care and death benefits, enrolled in a study to record the natural history of syphilis in hopes of justifying treatment programs for blacks. Many subjects progressed through the full course of untreated syphilis, ultimately ending in death. Participants entered this unethical research experiment without informed consent. Contemporary African Americans continue to harbor fear and mistrust of formal medical services and research because of the atrocities of the Tuskegee experiment.

Stigma and stereotypes associated with mental health illness are important obstacles for the elderly accessing mental health services. Compared with younger adults, older adults more often have negative attitudes toward mental health and mental health providers (Currin et al. 1998; Lundervold and Young 1992). Many older adults prefer to obtain mental health services from primary care providers (Waxman et al. 1984). Older African Americans, compared with white older adults, hold even more negative attitudes toward seeking mental health treatment (Snowden 2001). Compared with white elders, African American elders report that they are more likely to experience stigma associated with mental illness within their communities (Cooper-Patrick et al. 1997).

LITERATURE REVIEW OF PSYCHIATRIC DISORDERS IN THE AFRICAN AMERICAN POPULATION

Mental illnesses are common in the United States. One in six (44.7 million) U.S. adults lives with a mental illness (National Institute of Mental Health 2017). The conditions most commonly reported among older adults are anxiety and mood disorders (e.g., depression) (Hybels and Blazer 2015). Mental health issues are often cited as precipitating factors in cases of suicide. Older men have the highest suicide rate of any age group (Centers for Disease Control and Prevention 2017). Substance abuse, particularly of alcohol and prescription drugs, among adults 60 years and older is one of the fastest-growing health problems facing the country (Substance Abuse and Mental Health Services Administration 2011). In the following sections, I discuss epidemiology, diagnosis, and treatment of the following disorders among African American older adults: depression, bipolar disorder, substance use disorders, psychotic disorders, and neurocognitive disorders.

DEPRESSION

Depression is associated with increased disability, chronic medical conditions, and stressful life events. The disorder places a significant burden on patients, their communities, the economy, and the health care system (Gum et al. 2009; Richardson et al. 2012).

Prevalence

Racial and ethnic minority older adults experience more psychological distress compared with whites as a result of exposure to and/or experience with chronic stressors such as racism, discrimination, poverty, and violence (Cole and Dendukuri 2003; U.S. Department of Health and Human Services 2001). However, research on prevalence and symptom profiles of major depressive disorder among older African Americans is conflicting. Some studies reported older whites to have higher depression prevalence rates than African Americans (Aranda et al. 2012; Steffens et al. 2009; Woodward et al. 2012), whereas others reported no significant racial differences (Byers et al. 2010; Fyffe et al. 2004).

Comorbid Medical Conditions

The rate of functional impairment and chronic illnesses increases with age, placing older adults at greater risk for depression (Djernes et al. 1998; Mezuk et al. 2012). Depressive symptoms contribute to increasing disability, worsening physical illnesses, greater risk of developing additional medical conditions, and mortality (Cole and Dendukuri 2003; Unützer et al. 2002). However, when compared with medically compromised older whites, older African Americans with greater functional impairments had significantly lower levels of depressive symptoms (Cummings et al. 2003). The investigators attributed these results to greater religious involvement among African Americans, but there has been little research investigating the interrelationship of ethnicity, spirituality, depression, and medical comorbidity. Although there is a robust body of research on the impact of depression on older adults in general, far fewer studies have examined the effect of late-life depression on the health and well-being of African American older adults. The limited research on the diagnosis and treatment of depression in older

African Americans results in a significant gap in epidemiological and clinical knowledge about this population (Pickett et al. 2013).

Cultural Concepts of Distress

DSM-5 (American Psychiatric Association 2013) has significantly redefined the culture-bound syndromes previously outlined in DSM-IV-TR (American Psychiatric Association 2000) as *cultural concepts of distress*. DSM-5 articulates the dynamic interaction of culture and the expression of emotional distress in terms of three distinct concepts:

1. *Cultural syndromes*—"clusters of symptoms and attributions that tend to co-occur among individuals in specific cultural groups, communities, or contexts...that are recognized locally as coherent patterns of experience" (DSM-5, p. 758)
2. *Cultural idioms of distress*—"ways of expressing distress that may not involve specific symptoms or syndromes, but that provide collective, shared ways of experiencing and talking about personal or social concerns" (DSM-5, p. 758)
3. *Cultural explanations of distress* or *perceived causes*—"labels, attributions, or features of an explanatory model that indicate culturally recognized meaning or etiology for symptoms, illness, or distress" (DSM-5, p. 758)

In DSM-5, the number of culture-bound syndromes has been reduced from 25 to 9, and the clinical entities previously associated with African American culture (falling-out, spell, and rootwork) have been eliminated.

Treatment

Pharmacotherapy

Since the 1990s, there has been expanded public acceptance of psychopharmacological interventions for depression (Akincigil et al. 2012), greater awareness of depression, and greater willingness to seek professional help (Akincigil et al. 2012; Mojtabai 2008). However, there still are significant disparities in depression care among African American older adults compared with white older adults. Ethnic differences in depression diagnosis and treatment have been associated with provider factors, patient factors, and the treatment setting.

Provider factors.   Primary care physicians provide the majority of care for late-life depression, especially for African American elders (Burnett-Zeigler et al. 2014; Snowden and Pingitore 2002). Numerous studies outline the discriminatory behavior of providers (Bailey et al. 2011; Balsa and McGuire 2003; Institute of Medicine 2002), which contributes to ethnic disparities in depression. Primary care physicians are less likely to diagnose or treat depression in African American older adults compared with white older adults (Akincigil et al. 2012; Gallo et al. 2005). Primary care physicians often have limited mental health training and may have difficulty recognizing depressive symptoms in older African Americans (Borowsky et al. 2000; Brown et al. 1999). Numerous studies suggest that older African Americans are less likely to receive depression care and appropriate pharmacological interventions in the primary care setting (Alegría et al. 2009; Conner et al. 2010c; Unützer et al. 2003). Studies suggest that primary care physicians conduct shorter outpatient sessions (Das et al. 2006; Olfson et al. 2009) and provide fewer rapport-building statements when discussing depression care with African American patients than they do with white patients (Ghods et al. 2008; Hunt et al. 2013).

Providers are less likely to prescribe antidepressants to older African Americans than to other ethnic elders (Pickett et al. 2012, 2014). Studies suggest that primary care providers are also less likely to prescribe the most up-to-date depression treatment interventions for African American elders (González et al. 2008; Hall et al. 2015; Pickett et al. 2012). A study of primary care physicians elucidated their reasons for choosing not to prescribe antidepressant treatment for African American elders: Some physicians felt that the patients' depressive symptoms were too mild to warrant treatment with antidepressants (Gallo et al. 2005). Others believed that African Americans would be more reluctant than white patients to accept the diagnosis of depression or medication treatments (Cooper et al. 2003b; Gallo et al. 2005).

Patient factors. African Americans with depression are less likely to be in treatment (Conner et al. 2010c, 2010b; Das et al. 2006) and more likely to terminate treatment prematurely (Brown and Palenchar 2004). Numerous illness beliefs about depression negatively affect African American elders' participation in pharmacological treatments (Choi and Gonzalez 2005; Egede 2002). African American elders may be especially concerned about antidepressant medication side effects and the perceived addictive potential of these agents (Cooper et al. 2000). They may believe that depression is the result of personal weakness or improper lifestyle (e.g., too much work, too much worry, not being pious enough) (Kaskow et al. 2011; Shellman et al. 2007). Others report less family and community support helping them access mental health services (Joo et al. 2011). Stigma and shame about mental illness significantly contribute to the negative attitudes that African Americans express about depression (Brown et al. 2010; Choi and Gonzalez 2005; Conner et al. 2010c).

African American elders have experienced a lifetime of discrimination, racism, and prejudice, but they have learned to survive despite these oppressive circumstances (Conner et al. 2010c, 2010b). These stressful life experiences have negatively affected African Americans' attitudes about mental illness and seeking professional mental health treatment. Many African American elders prefer to keep their mental health status private and resist talking to those outside their community. They are more likely to seek emotional support from their informal support networks, the church, and primary care physicians (Administration on Aging 2001; Snowden 2001). The literature suggests that African American older adults do not believe mainstream mental health services will be effective, delay professional help seeking, and use culturally endorsed coping strategies for dealing with depression (Conner et al. 2010b).

African American older adults report limited trust in mental health service providers, attend fewer psychotherapy sessions (Connolly Gibbons et al. 2011), and have negative attitudes toward psychotherapy (Thompson et al. 2004). Many African Americans believe that psychotherapists lack adequate knowledge of African American history, life experience, and culture. They fear misdiagnosis, labeling, and brainwashing (Thompson et al. 2004). Others believe that mental health clinicians view all African Americans as crazy and that clinicians are prone to labeling strong expressions of emotion as illness (Thompson et al. 2004).

Older African Americans with depression perceive and experience a great deal of stigma that adversely affects their treatment-seeking attitudes and behaviors (Brown et al. 2010; Conner et al. 2010c, 2010a). Often, these patients and their families have limited knowledge about late-life depression (Conner et al. 2010a). They may consider depressive symptoms a normal part of the aging process and just another part of the African American experience (Conner et al. 2010a). Others may feel that it is a weakness to seek professional mental health treatment and that they should be able to handle depressive symptoms on their own (Conner et al. 2010a). African American women may be particularly prone to believe that they need to be strong in light of significant stress, loss, and depression (Beauboeuf-Lafontant 2007).

Treatment setting.   Some researchers have postulated that ethnic differences in pharmacokinetics may explain why African American adults may be less responsive to treatment with selective serotonin reuptake inhibitors (Friedman et al. 2009; Mrazek et al. 2009). Mrazek et al. suggested that ethnic differences in the gene regulating the serotonin transporter contribute to African Americans' poorer response to treatment with citalopram, but other authors found no ethnic differences in antidepressant efficacy (Lester et al. 2010).

Other treatment setting factors that contribute to ethnic disparities in care include poor access to health care services, limited insurance coverage for mental health treatment, and geographic differences in the availability of mental health interventions (Baicker and Chandra 2004; Bailey et al. 2011; Institute of Medicine 2002). Emergency departments and primary care clinics, where many African American older adults are treated, are particularly vulnerable to providing fragmented, inadequate care for mental health disorders (Bailey et al. 2011).

Psychotherapy

Research on older African Americans' attitudes to psychotherapy has produced contradictory results. Some studies indicated that African American older adults report limited trust in mental health service providers, attend fewer psychotherapy sessions (Connolly Gibbons et al. 2011), and have negative attitudes toward psychotherapy (Thompson et al. 2004). These issues are heightened when patients are seeing a clinician from a different racial or ethnic group or a younger clinician (Conner et al. 2010c; 2010a). In addition, African American older adults may be more reluctant to seek referrals from friends and family (Joo et al. 2011). Other authors report no racial differences in older adults regarding their attitude toward counseling or psychotherapy (Kasckow et al. 2011). Alvidrez and Arcán (2002) reported a significant improvement in psychotherapy attendance when African Americans received psychoeducation about treatment.

Religious beliefs and spiritual practices strongly influence African Americans' participation in mental health treatment. Faith and spirituality play vital roles in depression risk, course, and treatment in older African Americans (Jimenez et al. 2013). Attending religious services regularly significantly reduces the odds of a lifetime mood disorder (Givens et al. 2007). Many African American older adults have strong faith in God and in the power of religion to heal depression. Church-based social support may be particularly important for older African Americans given their extremely high rates of religious service attendance and overall religious participation (Taylor et al. 2007). Taylor et al. underscored the importance of psychiatrists in forging collaborative relationships with the spiritual community to promote greater engagement of older African Americans in treatment. Psychiatrists were encouraged to more actively incorporate spirituality into their treatment approaches (Givens et al. 2007; Wittink et al. 2009).

Provider factors and psychotherapy.   Primary care physicians provide the majority of later-life depression treatment, particularly for African Americans (Luber et al. 2001; Neighbors et al. 2008). Underdiagnosis of depression in African Americans compared with whites in primary care settings is a significant barrier to these patients receiving mental health treatment in a timely fashion (Borowsky et al. 2000).

Akincigil et al. (2012) reported that only 51% of African American elders with depression received antidepressants, and only 18% received psychotherapy. Declining rates of psychotherapy among older adults may reflect managed care's increasing constraints on access to services (Mechanic et al. 1999). Reduced access to psychotherapy is particularly problematic for African American older adults, who report greater preference for counseling over pharmacotherapy (Cooper et al. 2003a; Givens et al. 2007).

Treatment setting and psychotherapy.   Although community- and home-based nonpharmacological depression treatment interventions show promising results, there has been little research on the efficacy and cultural relevance of these psychotherapeutic approaches for older African Americans (Casado et al. 2008; Gitlin et al. 2013; Klug et al. 2010; Quitano et al. 2007). Studies report ethnic differences in depression treatment acceptability, with African Americans expressing lower acceptability of antidepressant medication (Cooper et al. 2003a), greater preference for counseling (Dwight-Johnson et al. 2000), and more interest in counseling from clergy (Blank et al. 2002) compared with whites. Several studies have recommended integrating time-limited behavioral interventions with home-based and trusted community-based service organizations (e.g., senior centers) (Gitlin et al. 2013). African American elders may view this collaborative interagency approach as a more culturally acceptable, accessible treatment option (Gitlin 2014; Gitlin et al. 2013).

Health policy research suggests that collaborative care interventions focused on depression management in older adults can reduce disparities and improve medical and mental health outcomes in African American older adults (Areán et al. 2005; Miranda et al. 2003). However, this treatment model may not be viable because public and private sector health care organizations have reduced the number of visits, duration of treatment, and amount of reimbursement per visit for psychotherapy (Olfson et al. 2002).

Clinical Course and Outcomes

Several studies have suggested that compared with older whites, older African Americans were more persistently depressed (Breslau et al. 2009;

Lenze et al. 2005) and had higher rates of depressive symptoms and recurrent major depressive disorder (González et al. 2010). Studies of community-dwelling older adults suggested that the variables most predictive of depression outcomes are older age, external locus of control, chronic somatic illness, baseline depression, and functional status (Licht-Strunk et al. 2009). In general, the adverse outcomes most often associated with untreated depression included increased all-cause mortality, suicide, coronary heart disease, increased physical health problems, and functional disability (Unützer et al. 2002; Wulsin and Singal 2003). However, none of these studies examined factors associated with depression outcomes in relation to the experiences of older African Americans.

BIPOLAR DISORDER

Prevalence

Prevalence rates of bipolar disorder are similar across ethnic and racial groups. However, some authors reported that patients with bipolar disorder who are members of racial or ethnic minority groups continue to receive less intensive specialized mental health treatment than do white patients (Gonzalez et al. 2007).

Pharmacotherapy

Research on pharmacotherapy of bipolar disorder reveals limited information on ethnic differences in medication response. Studies of the pharmacodynamics of lithium therapy suggest that compared with whites, African Americans develop a higher lithium red blood cell–to-plasma ratio and also report more side effects (Strickland et al. 1995). Several authors suggested that African Americans may benefit from treatment with lower doses of lithium to promote better tolerability (Strickland et al. 1993, 1995). There are no published randomized controlled trials examining the prevalence of side effects and medication efficacy for other mood-stabilizing agents among African Americans.

SUBSTANCE USE DISORDERS

Prevalence

The population of people ages 65 and older increased from 36.6 million in 2005 to 47.8 million in 2015 (a 30% increase), and the number of older adults is projected to more than double to 98 million in 2060 (Administration on Aging 2016). A study conducted by the Substance Abuse and Mental Health Services Administration in 2009 revealed that abuse of illicit drugs by older adults is on the rise (Substance Abuse and Mental Health Services Administration 2010). This same study also revealed dramatic increases in illicit drug use in older adults, including nonmedical use of prescription drugs among women ages 60–64 years. Illicit drug use among adults age 50 or older is projected to increase from 2.2% to 3.1% between 2001 and 2020 (Colliver et al. 2006), and the number of older Americans with substance use disorder is expected to rise from 2.8 million in 2002–2006 to 5.7 million by 2020 (Wu and Blazer 2011). Overall, alcohol was the most frequently reported primary substance of abuse for persons age 50 and older. Opioids were the second most commonly reported primary substance of abuse, reported most frequently by individuals ages 50–59.

Early-Onset Versus Late-Onset Substance Use

Older adults with a substance use disorder are categorized as early-onset or late-onset users. Among early-onset users, substance abuse develops before age 65. In these individuals, the incidence of psychiatric and physical problems tends to be higher than in their late-onset counterparts. In late-onset substance abusers, addictive behaviors are often thought to develop subsequent to stressful life situations such as the losses that commonly occur with aging (e.g., death of a partner, changes in living situation, retirement, social isolation). These individuals typically experience fewer physical and mental health problems than do early-onset abusers (Brennan and Moos 1996).

Alcohol Use Disorder

Compared with whites, African Americans report higher rates of abstention from alcohol (Galvan and Caetano 2003; Substance Abuse and Mental Health Services Administration 2010, 2011). However, African Americans who do engage in drinking behaviors appear to be at a comparable and, at times, higher risk for experiencing alcohol-related problems (Galvan and Caetano 2003; Jones-Webb 1998), negative social consequences from drinking (Mulia et al. 2009), higher rates of alcohol-related illness and injuries (Greenfield 2001; Yoon et al. 2001), and higher rates of moderate to severe alcohol use disorders (Caetano 1997; Mulia et al. 2009) as compared with whites. Studies of mixed-age populations suggest that there are ethnic differences in utilization of alcohol treatment programs (Chartier and Caetano 2011). African Americans are less likely than whites to seek alcohol treatment and/or see a substance abuse health professional (Chartier and Caetano 2011). These ethnic differences in service utilization may be associated with access barriers such as limited disposable income or inadequate insurance coverage.

Psychosocial Factors

Psychosocial factors that negatively affect treatment completion rates among African American patients are greater duration of drug use before admission to treatment programs and homelessness. Compared with white patients, African Americans enter substance use treatment with more health, mental health, and social problems, which can contribute to reduced treatment completion (Marsh et al. 2009). The cumulative effect of the severity of drug use and greater prevalence of mental health problems and homelessness place African Americans and other minorities at a disadvantage in terms of successful participation in a demanding, structured treatment program (Grella and Stein 2006; Niv et al. 2009). More research is needed to elucidate the patient, provider, and treatment setting factors that affect substance use disorder treatment referral and admission and adherence rates, particularly for African American older adults.

PSYCHOTIC DISORDERS

Treated prevalence studies consistently find that African Americans are more likely than whites to be diagnosed with schizophrenia (Blow et al. 2004; Lawson et al. 1994) and less likely to receive psychotic affective and bipolar diagnoses (Strawkowsky et al. 2003). Several authors have reported that African Americans are often misdiagnosed with schizophrenia, which contributes to unnecessary exposure to neuroleptic treatment and inadequate and inappropriate treatment (Eack et al. 2012; McEvoy et al. 2005). Misdiagnosis of psychotic disorder may be due to numerous factors, including clinician bias, misinterpretation of psychotic symptoms, culturally biased diagnostic tools, and patient-clinician sociocultural differences (U.S. Department of Health and Human Services 2001). Therefore, it is critical that all elderly patients, especially African American older adults, be carefully evaluated because their previous diagnoses may not be correct.

The relationship between ethnicity and psychopharmacological interventions for psychiatric disorders is an important clinical issue for

African American older adults. In addition, studies suggest that African American patients with psychotic disorders may be more significantly impacted by provider factors and treatment setting issues than are white patients.

Provider Factors

Providers disproportionally diagnose African American psychiatric patients with schizophrenia compared with white patients and may minimize affective symptoms. Although African Americans can respond to similar medication doses as those given to whites, African Americans receive higher doses of antipsychotics despite evidence that they are more vulnerable to side effects (Lawson 2008). Some authors suggest that African Americans are treated with higher doses of antipsychotics because of (usually non–African American) therapists' lack of engagement with this patient population (Segal et al. 1996). Ethnic differences in antipsychotic treatment also may be related to the social perception that African Americans are more violent (Lawson 2008). Physicians are more likely to prescribe depot antipsychotics to African Americans but are less likely to prescribe second-generation antipsychotics (Aggarwal et al. 2012; Arnold et al. 2004; Brown et al. 2014; Puyat et al. 2013).

Treatment Factors

African American older adults are at increased risk for developing medication-induced movement disorders (e.g., tardive dyskinesia) from treatment with both first- and second-generation antipsychotics (Tenback et al. 2009; Woerner et al. 2011). Higher rates of antipsychotic-induced movement disorders among African Americans may be due to their more frequent exposure to high doses of antipsychotics (Lindamer et al. 1999). Other authors suggest that genetically determined metabolic differences may contribute to the higher rates of medication-induced movement disorders in this patient population (Bradford 2002; Shen et al. 2007). Compared with whites, African Americans more often have the cytochrome P450 (CYP) 2D6 allelic variants *CYP2D6*10* and *CYP2D6*17*, both of which are associated with decreased catabolic efficiency of antipsychotic medications (Shen et al. 2007).

Long-term treatment with atypical antipsychotic drugs can induce metabolic syndrome (Fujimoto et al. 1995; Komossa et al. 2010; Stauffer et al. 2010). Because African Americans are at increased risk of developing diabetes and obesity, antipsychotic treatment can greatly increase their odds of developing these disorders. Close monitoring and collaboration with primary care providers are critical in preventing the emergence of metabolic syndrome among African American older adults treated with antipsychotics.

Medication outcome literature in schizophrenia across racial or ethnic groups is sparse and produces inconsistent findings. The Clinical Antipsychotic Trials of Intervention Effectiveness (CATIE) examined race/ethnicity outcomes for study discontinuation and secondary outcomes (Arnold et al. 2013). African Americans experienced fewer side effects than whites but were more likely to drop out of the study after the first phase. Increased discontinuation rates were thought to be driven by research burden, personal issues, and unspecified loss to follow-up (Arnold et al. 2013).

NEUROCOGNITIVE DISORDERS

Cognitive impairment in older adults occurs for a variety of reasons, including medication side effects; metabolic and/or endocrine derangements; and delirium due to medical illness, depression, or dementia. Alzheimer's disease (AD) is a frequent cause of cognitive decline. Even after adjusting for education and other potentially confounding variables, African Americans have approximately a 2.5-fold higher risk than whites for both early-onset and late-onset Alzheimer's disease (Chen and Panegyres 2016; Demirovic et al. 2003; Griffith et al. 2006; Tang et al. 2001). However, clinical data on the treatment of African Americans with Alzheimer's disease and related disorders are scarce. For older African Americans, who comprise one of the fastest-growing minority groups, the diagnosis of AD comes at more advanced stages, when care is costlier and outcomes from pharmacological and nonpharmacological interventions are less promising (Lilienfeld and Perl 1994; Stephenson 2001).

Treatment

African American older adults have been underrepresented in clinical trials of pharmacological interventions for dementia, including studies of cholinesterase inhibitors. In an open-label study, Griffith et al. (2006) concluded that donepezil is effective and safe in treating African Americans with mild to moderate AD. The authors recommended that future studies should be randomized placebo-controlled trials, which would allow more rigorous evaluation of treatment effects in minority elders.

Numerous authors report that African Americans are substantially less likely than non-Hispanic whites to receive an acetylcholinesterase inhibitor or memantine even after controlling for several demographic variables (Hernandez et al. 2010; Kalkonde et al. 2009; Mehta et al. 2005). Causes for treatment disparities among African American elders can be divided into three factors: patient factors, provider factors, and treatment setting.

Patient Factors

Patients' culture-bound explanatory models of disease significantly affect their engagement in treatment (Hernandez et al. 2010). African American elders and their families have a greater tendency to perceive dementia as a natural part of aging, and they may be unaware of or may minimize the symptoms that emerge in the earlier stages of the disease (Connell et al. 2007; Hipps et al. 2003). Minority patients may also be wary of newer medications and treatment approaches, reflecting a need for better patient education. Media may also play a role, reflecting and propagating barriers, as seen in the low prioritization of pharmaceutical advertising in black- versus white-oriented media (Omonuwa 2001).

Provider Factors

Provider practices that contribute to treatment disparities for African American elders include subtle bias in community health care systems, underdiagnosis of dementia, and reluctance to prescribe newer medications to minority patients (Hernandez et al. 2010).

Treatment Setting

Treatment setting factors that adversely affect African American older adults include inadequate insurance coverage, limited pharmacy access to anticholinesterase inhibitors or memantine, limited availability and adequacy of dementia assessment resources, and reduced access to primary care physicians (Hernandez et al. 2010).

Caregiver Coping Strategies

Numerous studies have found that African American caregivers of patients with dementia report less anxiety (Bekhet 2015; Haley et al. 1995), depression (Bekhet 2015; Clay et al. 2008), and hostility (Bekhet 2015; Haley et al. 1995) than do white caregivers. Evidence suggests that African American caregivers demonstrate higher levels of resourcefulness, positive cognitions, and psychological well-being (Bekhet 2015) when compared with white caregivers. These social resourcefulness skills may act as buffers against the anxiety, depression, and hostility associated with caregiver stress (Bekhet 2015). Some authors suggest that social resourcefulness skills should be taught to caregivers. This skills training might include helping caregivers rely on family and friends, exchanging ideas with other caregivers, and seeking professional help when appropriate (Bekhet 2015). Some investigators have suggested teaching coping strategies, such as reframing a difficult situation in a positive way and interrupting negative thoughts with distraction and relaxation techniques (Bekhet 2015; Bekhet and Zauszniewski 2013).

Health Beliefs and Public Education

Connell et al. (2007) and Mahoney et al. (2005) reported that compared with white respondents, African Americans were significantly more likely to believe that AD is a normal part of aging and showed a greater lack of awareness of early signs of AD (Connell et al. 2007). Overall, these results suggest that misconceptions about AD remain among large segments of the African American population, that AD remains a source of significant concern, and that continued efforts are needed to educate the public about this disease (Connell et al. 2007). Several authors advocate that public education outreach about dementia should focus on efforts, particularly among racially and ethnically diverse groups, to increase awareness that Alzheimer's disease is not part of normal aging. There is a growing need for the development of successful, culturally sensitive educational interventions for minority caregivers and people affected directly by the disease (Teri et al. 2003). These educational interventions may focus on informing African American elders and their families about risk-reduction strategies to prevent AD and pharmacological, behavioral, and social approaches to help manage the disease and improve quality of life (Connell et al. 2007).

End-of-Life Care

Research is limited on the process by which end-of-life treatment decisions are made by African American family caregivers. Interventions at the end of life for people with dementia from some ethnic minorities, particularly African Americans, were found to be different from whites in that they were less likely to use hospice services (Campbell et al. 2011; Crawley et al. 2000), less likely to have a do-not-resuscitate order (Burgio et al. 2016), and less likely to have advance directives (Waite et al. 2013; Zaide et al. 2013). Studies of end-of-life care for people without dementia from ethnic minorities have shown a tendency for African Americans and other ethnic minorities to choose more aggressive end-of-life care (Degenholtz et al. 2002; Kwak and Haley 2005). Although the qualitative evidence suggests that attitudes toward end-of-life care are more similar than different between African Americans and whites, two studies found that physician characteristics, including the ethnicity of the physician, and the proportion of ethnic minority residents in the facility were important factors (Krakauer et al. 2002; Kwak and Haley 2005). Other factors that may contribute to the greater use of life-sustaining treatments in ethnic minority groups (particularly African Americans) include mistrust of medical service providers associated with fears of undertreatment, lack of knowledge or information, and differing cultural evaluations of the risks and benefits of artificial nutrition and hydration (Krakauer et al. 2002; Kwak and Haley 2005).

Other authors have concluded that health literacy and not race is an independent predictor of end-of-life preferences (Volandes et al. 2008). Volandes et al. compared subjects' preferences after hearing a verbal description of advanced dementia and again after viewing a video of a patient with dementia, and the results suggested that clinical practice and research relating to end-of-life preferences may need to focus on a patient education model incorporating the use of decision aids such as video to ensure informed decision making.

African American and Hispanic nursing home residents with severe dementia are less likely to have do-not-hospitalize orders than are white residents (Monroe and Carter 2010). Studies reported that less than 9% of African Americans have made advance care plans, as opposed to 18%–30% of whites (Gerst and Burr 2008; Ghiotti 2009). Although African Americans are three times more likely than whites to be diagnosed with dementia, they disproportionately receive less dementia care and education (Daaleman et al. 2008; Waters 2000). Consequently, most African Americans with dementia must rely on family members to make their decisions about critical end-of-life treatment, such as cardiopulmonary resuscitation, mechanical ventilation, and tube feeding (Wang et al. 2000). In order for caregivers to make informed end-of-life treatment decisions for cognitively impaired relatives, they must be knowledgeable about the consequences and trajectory of the disease. In addition, caregivers will become better equipped to make these choices in advance when they are provided knowledge, such as benefits and risks and alternative treatments.

KEY POINTS

- The number of older African Americans in the United States will likely increase to 12 million by 2060, making them the second-largest segment of the ethnic minority older adult population.

- African American older adults often receive financial, instrumental, and emotional support from a broad social network consisting of family members and fictive kin.
- Among African American elderly, significant health care disparities exist in both access to care and treatment for a variety of mental health conditions, including depression, serious mental illness, and neurocognitive disorders.
- Knowledge of historical and cultural contexts is necessary to design and target interventions to promote health-seeking behaviors and decrease health care disparities for African American older adults.
- Mental health care disparities of African American older adults are highly influenced by the dynamic interaction between patient beliefs and knowledge, treatment setting factors, and physician practice patterns.
- Future research is needed in the diagnosis and treatment interventions for specific psychiatric disorders in African American older adults (e.g., bipolar disorder, substance use disorders, psychotic disorders).

QUESTIONS FOR FURTHER THOUGHT

1. West African health traditions reflect a holistic ideology in which good health is the result of a harmonious relationship with nature and man and disease is classified under all of the following headings except

    A. Natural.
    B. Occult.
    C. Spiritual.
    D. Traditional.

2. True or False: The U.S. Public Health Service's Tuskegee Study of Untreated Syphilis enrolled 600 African Americans, promising free health care and death benefits, but resulted in many subjects progressing through the full course of untreated syphilis, ultimately ending in their death.

3. True or False: Older African Americans are more likely than older whites to perceive cognitive impairment as a normal part of aging.

4. Compared with white caregivers of older adults with neurocognitive impairment, African American caregivers are more likely to demonstrate which of the following?

   A. Depression.
   B. Anxiety.
   C. Hostility.
   D. Resourcefulness.

SUGGESTED READINGS AND WEBSITES

Fabre G, O'Meally R (eds): History and Memory in African-American Culture. New York, Oxford University Press, 1994

National Museum of African American History and Culture: https:// nmaahc.si.edu

Stanford School of Medicine: Health and Healthcare of African American Older Adults. Stanford, CA, Stanford School of Medicine. Available at: https://geriatrics.stanford.edu/ethnomed/african_american.html.

Van Deburg WL: Black Camelot: African-American Culture Heroes in Their Times, 1960–1980. Chicago, IL, University of Chicago Press, 2008

REFERENCES

Administration on Aging: Older Adults and Mental Health: Issues and Opportunities. Washington, DC, U.S. Department of Health and Human Services, January 2001. Available at: www.public-health.uiowa.edu/icmha/training/documents/Older-Adults-and-Mental-Health-2001.pdf. Accessed May 4, 2018.

Administration on Aging: A Profile of Older Americans: 2016. Washington, DC, U.S. Department of Health and Human Services, 2016. Available at: www.giaging.org/documents/A_Profile_of_Older_Americans__2016.pdf. Accessed: May 4, 2018.

Administration for Community Living: Minority Aging. Washington, DC, Administration for Community Living, September 2017. Available at: www.acl.gov/aging-and-disability-in-america/data-and-research/minority-aging. Accessed December 23, 2017.

Aggarwal NK, Rosenheck RA, Woods SW, et al: Race and long-acting antipsychotic prescription at a community mental health center: a retrospective chart review. J Clin Psychiatry 73(4):513–517, 2012 22579151

Akincigil A, Olfson M, Siegel M, et al: Racial and ethnic disparities in depression care in community-dwelling elderly in the United States. Am J Public Health 102(2):319–328, 2012 22390446

Alegría M, Pescosolido B, Canino G: A socio-cultural framework for mental health and substance abuse service disparities, in Kaplan and Sadock's Comprehensive Textbook of Psychiatry, 9th Edition, Volume 2. Edited by Sadock BJ, Sadock VA, Ruiz P. Philadelphia, PA, Wolters Kluwer Health/ Lippincott Williams & Wilkins, 2009, pp 4370–4379

Alvidrez J, Areán PA: Physician willingness to refer older depressed patients for psychotherapy. Int J Psychiatry Med 32(1):21–35, 2002 12075914

American Psychiatric Association: Diagnostic and Statistical Manual of Mental Disorders, 4th Edition, Text Revision. Washington, DC, American Psychiatric Association, 2000

American Psychiatric Association: Diagnostic and Statistical Manual of Mental Disorders, 5th Edition. Arlington, VA, American Psychiatric Association, 2013

Aranda M, Chae DH, Lincoln KD, et al: Demographic correlates of DSM-IV major depressive disorder among older African Americans, black Caribbeans, and non-Hispanic whites: results from the National Survey of American Life. Int J Geriatr Psychiatry 27(9):940–947, 2012 22038674

Areán PA, Ayalon L, Hunkeler E, et al.; IMPACT Investigators: Improving depression care for older, minority patients in primary care. Med Care 43(4):381–390, 2005 15778641

Arnold JG, Miller AL, Cañive JM, et al: Comparison of outcomes for African Americans, Hispanics, and non-Hispanic whites in the CATIE study. Psychiatr Serv 64(6):570–578, 2013 23494108

Arnold LM, Strakowski SM, Schwiers ML, et al: Sex, ethnicity, and antipsychotic medication use in patients with psychosis. Schizophr Res 66(2–3):169–175, 2004 15061250

Baicker K, Chandra A: Medicare spending, the physician workforce, and beneficiaries' quality of care. Health Aff (Millwood) (suppl Web exclusives):W4–184–197, 2004 15451981

Bailey RK, Patel M, Barker NC, et al: Major depressive disorder in the African American population. J Natl Med Assoc 103(7):548–557, 2011 21999029

Balsa AI, McGuire TG: Prejudice, clinical uncertainty and stereotyping as sources of health disparities. J Health Econ 22(1):89–116, 2003 12564719

Beauboeuf-Lafontant T: You have to show strength: an exploration of gender, race and depression. Gend Soc 21:28–51, 2007

Becker G, Beyene Y, Newsom E, et al: Creating continuity through mutual assistance: intergenerational reciprocity in four ethnic groups. J Gerontol B Psychol Sci Soc Sci 58(3):S151–S159, 2003 12730316

Bekhet AK: Resourcefulness in African American and Caucasian American caregivers of persons with dementia: associations with perceived burden, depression, anxiety, positive cognitions, and psychological well-being. Perspect Psychiatr Care 51(4):285–294, 2015 25495263

Bekhet AK, Zauszniewski JA: Measuring use of positive thinking skills: psychometric testing of a new scale. West J Nurs Res 35(8):1074–1093, 2013 23509101

Blank MB, Mahmood M, Fox JC, et al: Alternative mental health services: the role of the black church in the South. Am J Public Health 92(10):1668–1672, 2002 12356619

Blow FC, Zeber JE, McCarthy JF, et al: Ethnicity and diagnostic patterns in veterans with psychoses. Soc Psychiatry Psychiatr Epidemiol 39(10):841–851, 2004 15669666

Borowsky SJ, Rubenstein LV, Meredith LS, et al: Who is at risk of nondetection of mental health problems in primary care? J Gen Intern Med 15(6):381–388, 2000 10886472

Bradford LD: CYP2D6 allele frequency in European Caucasians, Asians, Africans and their descendants. Pharmacogenomics 3(2):229–243, 2002 11972444

Brennan PL, Moos RH: Late-life drinking behavior: the influence of personal characteristics, life context, and treatment. Alcohol Health Res World 20:197–204, 1996

Breslau J, Kender K, Su M, et al: Lifetime risk and persistence of psychiatric disorders across ethnic groups in the United States. Psychol Med 35(3):317–327, 2009 15841868

Brown C, Palenchar DR: Treatment of depression in African American primary care patients. African American Research Perspectives Spring–Summer:55–65, 2004

Brown C, Schulberg HC, Sacco D, et al: Effectiveness of treatments for major depression in primary medical care practice: a post hoc analysis of outcomes for African American and white patients. J Affect Disord 53(2):185–192, 1999 10360414

Brown C, Conner KO, Copeland VC, et al: Depression, stigma, race and treatment seeking behavior and Attitudes. J Community Psychol 38(3):350–368, 2010 21274407

Brown JD, Barrett A, Caffery E, et al: State and demographic variation in use of depot antipsychotics by Medicaid beneficiaries with schizophrenia. Psychiatr Serv 65(1):121–124, 2014 24382765

Burgio KL, Williams BR, Dionne-Odom JN, et al: Racial differences in processes of care at end of life in VA Medical Centers: planned secondary analysis of data from the BEACON trial. J Palliat Med 19(2):157–163, 2016 26840851

Burnett-Zeigler I, Kim HM, Chiang C, et al: The association between race and gender, treatment attitudes, and antidepressant treatment adherence. Int J Geriatr Psychiatry 29(2):169–177, 2014 23801324

Byers AL, Yaffe K, Covins KE, et al: High occurrence of mood and anxiety disorders among older adults: the National Comorbidity Survey Replication. Arch Gen Psychiatry 67(5):489–496, 2010 20439830

Caetano R: Prevalence, incidence and stability of drinking problems among whites, blacks and Hispanics: 1984–1992. J Stud Alcohol 58(6):565–572, 1997 9391915

Campbell CL, Williams IC, Orr T: Factors that impact end-of-life decision making in African Americans with advanced cancer. J Hosp Palliat Nurs 41(1):277–278 2011 23645999

Casado BL, Quijano LM, Stanley MA, et al: Healthy IDEAS: implementation of a depression program through community-based case management. Gerontologist 48(6):828–838, 2008 19139256

Centers for Disease Control and Prevention: Welcome to WISQARS. Atlanta, GA, Centers for Disease Control and Prevention, August 1, 2017. Available at: www.cdc.gov/injury/wisqars/index.html. Accessed December 23, 2017.

Chartier KG, Caetano R: Trends in alcohol services utilization from 1991–1992 to 2001–2002: ethnic group differences in the U.S. population. Alcohol Clin Exp Res 35(8):1485–1497, 2011 21575015

Chatters LM, Taylor RJ, Jayakody R: Fictive kinship relations in black extended families. J Comp Fam Stud 25:197–213, 1994

Chen HY, Panegyres PK: The role of ethnicity in Alzheimer's disease: findings from the C-PATH online data repository. J Alzheimers Dis 51(2):515–523, 2016 26890783

Choi NG, Gonzalez JM: Geriatric mental health clinician's perceptions of barriers and contributors to retention of older minorities in treatment: an exploratory study. Clin Gerontol 28:3–25, 2005

Clay OJ, Roth DL, Wadley VG, et al: Changes in social support and their impact on psychosocial outcome over a 5-year period for African American and white dementia caregivers. Int J Geriatr Psychiatry 23(8):857–862, 2008 18338341

Cole MG, Dendukuri N: Risk factors for depression among elderly community subjects: a systematic review and meta-analysis. Am J Psychiatry 160(6):1147–1156, 2003 12777274

Colliver JD, Compton WM, Gfroerer JC, Condon T: Projecting drug use among aging baby boomers in 2020. Ann Epidemiology 16(4):257–265 2006 16275134

Connell CM, Scott Roberts J, McLaughlin SJ: Public opinion about Alzheimer disease among blacks, Hispanics, and whites: results from a national survey. Alzheimer Dis Assoc Disord 21(3):232–240, 2007 17804956

Conner KO, Copeland VC, Grote N, et al: Barriers to treatment and culturally endorsed coping strategies among depressed African American older adults. Aging Ment Health 14(8):971–983, 2010a 21069603

Conner KO, Copeland VC, Grote NK, et al: Mental health treatment seeking among older adults with depression: the impact of stigma and race. Am J Geriatr Psychiatry 18(6):531–543, 2010b 20220602

Conner KO, Lee B, Mayers V, et al: Attitudes and beliefs about mental health among African American older adults suffering from depression. J Aging Stud 24(4):266–277, 2010c 21423819

Connolly Gibbons MB, Rothbard A, Farris KD, et al: Changes in psychotherapy utilization among consumers of services for major depressive disorder in the community mental health system. Adm Policy Ment Health 38(6):495–503, 2011 21298475

Cooper LA, Brown C, Vu HT, et al: Primary care patients' opinions regarding the importance of various aspects of care for depression. Gen Hosp Psychiatry 22(3):163–173, 2000 10880709

Cooper LA, Gonzales JJ, Gallo JJ, et al: The acceptability of treatment for depression among African-American, Hispanic, and white primary care patients. Med Care 41(4):479–489, 2003a 12665712

Cooper LA, Roter DL, Johnson RL, et al: Patient-centered communication, ratings of care, and concordance of patient and physician race. Ann Intern Med 139(11):907–915, 2003b 14644893

Cooper-Patrick L, Powe NR, Jenckes MW, et al: Identification of patient attitudes and preferences regarding treatment of depression. J Gen Intern Med 12(7):431–438, 1997 9229282

Covey HC: African American Slave Medicine: Herbal and Nonherbal Treatments. Lanham, MD, Lexington Books, 2007, p 5

Crawley L, Payne R, Bolden J, et al; Initiative to Improve Palliative and End-of-Life Care in the African American Community: Palliative and end-of-life care in the African American community. JAMA 284(19):2518–2521, 2000 11074786

Cummings SM, Neff JA, Husaini BA: Functional impairment as a predictor of depressive symptomatology: the role of race, religiosity, and social support. Health Soc Work 28(1):23–32, 2003 12621930

Currin B, Hayslip B, Schneider W, et al: Cohort differences in attitudes toward mental health services among older persons. Psychotherapy 35(4):506–518, 1998

Daaleman TP, Emmett CP, Dobbs D, et al: An exploratory study of advance care planning in seriously ill African-American elders. J Natl Med Assoc 100(12):1457–1462, 2008 19110915

Das AK, Olfson M, McCurtis HL et al: Depression in African Americans: breaking barriers to detection and treatment. J Fam Pract 55(1):30–39, 2006 16388764

Degenholtz HB, Arnold RA, Meisel A, et al: Persistence of racial disparities in advance care plan documents among nursing home residents. J Am Geriatr Soc 50(2):378–381, 2002 12028224

Demirovic J, Prineas R, Loewenstein D, et al: Prevalence of dementia in three ethnic groups: the South Florida program on aging and health. Ann Epidemiol 13(6):472–478, 2003 12875807

DeNavas-Walt C, Proctor BD: Income and Poverty in the United States: 2014. Suitland, MD, U.S. Census Bureau, 2015. Available at: www.census.gov/content/dam/Census/library/publications/2015/demo/p60-252.pdf. Accessed: May 4, 2018.

Djernes JK, Gulmann NC, Abelskov KE, et al: Psychopathologic and functional outcome in the treatment of elderly inpatients with depressive disorders, dementia, delirium and psychoses. Int Psychogeriatr 10(1):71–83, 1998 9629526

Dwight-Johnson M, Sherbourne CD, Liao D, et al: Treatment preferences among depressed primary care patients. J Gen Intern Med 15(8):527–534, 2000 10940143

Dunlop DD, Manheim LM, Song J, et al: Gender and ethnic/racial disparities in health care utilization among older adults. J Gerontol B Psychol Sci Soc Sci 57(4):S221–S233, 2002 12084792

Eack SM, Bahorik AL, Newhill CE, et al: Interviewer-perceived honesty as a mediator of racial disparities in the diagnosis of schizophrenia. Psychiatr Serv 63(9):875–880, 2012 22751938

Egede LE: Beliefs and attitudes of African Americans with type 2 diabetes toward depression. Diabetes Educ 28(2):258–268, 2002 11924303

Friedman ES, Wisniewski SR, Gilmer W, et al: Sociodemographic, clinical, and treatment characteristics associated with worsened depression during treatment with citalopram: results of the NIMH STAR(*)D trial. Depress Anxiety 26(7):612–621, 2009 19382183

Fujimoto WY, Bergstrom RW, Boyko EJ, et al: Susceptibility to development of central adiposity among populations. Obes Res 3(suppl 2):179S–186S, 1995 8581774

Fyffe DC, Sirey JA, Heo M, et al: Late-life depression among black and white elderly homecare patients. Am J Geriatr Psychiatry 12(5):531–535, 2004 15353393

Gallo JJ, Bogner HR, Morales KH, et al: Patient ethnicity and the identification and active management of depression in late life. Arch Intern Med 165(17):1962–1968, 2005 16186465

Galvan FH, Caetano R: Alcohol use and related problems among ethnic minorities in the United States. Alcohol Res Health 27(1):87–94, 2003 15301403

Gamble VN: Under the shadow of Tuskegee: African Americans and health care. Am J Public Health 87(11):1773–1778, 1997 9366634

Gerst K, Burr JA: Planning for end-of-life care: black-white differences in the completion of advance directives. Res Aging 30(4):428–449, 2008

Ghiotti C: The Dementia End of Life Care Project (DeLCaP): supporting families caring for people with late stage dementia at home. Dementia 8:349–361, 2009

Ghods BK, Roter DL, Ford DE, et al: Patient-physician communication in the primary care visits of African Americans and whites with depression. J Gen Intern Med 23(5):600–606, 2008 18264834

Gitlin LN: The role of community and home-based interventions in late life depression, in Richards CS, O'Hara MW. The Oxford Handbook of Depression and Comorbidity. London: Oxford University Press, 2014, pp 511–527

Gitlin LN, Harris LF, McCoy MC, et al: A home-based intervention to reduce depressive symptoms and improve quality of life in older African Americans: a randomized trial. Ann Intern Med 159(4):243–252, 2013 24026257

Givens JL, Katz IR, Bellamy S, et al: Stigma and the acceptability of depression treatments among African Americans and whites. J Gen Intern Med 22(9):1292–1297, 2007 17610120

González HM, Croghan T, West B, et al: Antidepressant use in black and white populations in the United States. Psychiatr Serv 59(10):1131–1138, 2008 18832498

González HM, Tarraf W, Whitfield K, Vega WA: The epidemiology of major depression and ethnicity in the United States. Psychiatr Res 44(15):1043–1051, 2010, 20537350

Gonzalez JM, Thompson P, Escamilla M, et al: Treatment characteristics and illness burden among European Americans, African Americans, and Latinos in the first 2,000 patients of the systematic treatment enhancement program for bipolar disorder. Psychopharmacol Bull 40(1):31–46, 2007 17285094

Greenfield TK: Health disparities in alcohol-related disorders, problems, and treatment use by minorities. FrontLines Linking Alcohol Services Research and Practice June:3–7, 2001

Grella CE, Stein JA: Impact of program services on treatment outcomes of patients with comorbid mental and substance use disorders. Psychiatr Serv 57(7):1007–1015, 2006 16816286

Griffith P, Lichtenberg P, Goldman R, et al: Safety and efficacy of donepezil in African Americans with mild-to-moderate Alzheimer's disease. J Natl Med Assoc 98(10):1590–1597, 2006 17052048

Gum AM, Petkus A, McDougal SJ, et al: Behavioral health needs and problem recognition by older adults receiving home-based aging services. Int J Geriatr Psychiatry 24(4):400–408, 2009 18836987

Haley WE, West CA, Wadley VG, et al: Psychological, social, and health impact of caregiving: a comparison of black and white dementia family caregivers and noncaregivers. Psychol Aging 10(4):540–552, 1995 8749581

Hall CA, Simon KM, Lenze EJ, et al: Depression remission rates among older black and white adults: analyses from the IRL-GREY trial. Psychiatr Serv 66(12):1303–1311, 2015 26278231

Hernandez S, McClendon MJ, Zhou XH, et al: Pharmacological treatment of Alzheimer's disease: effect of race and demographic variables. J Alzheimers Dis 19(2):665–672, 2010 20110610

Hines-Martin V, Usui W, Kim S, et al: A comparison of influences on attitudes towards mental health service use in an African-American and white community. J Natl Black Nurses Assoc 15(2):17–22, 2004 15853282

Hipps YG, Roberts JS, Farrer LA, et al: Differences between African Americans and whites in their attitudes toward genetic testing for Alzheimer's disease. Genet Test 7(1):39–44, 2003 12820701

Hunt J, Sullivan G, Chavira DA, et al: Race and beliefs about mental health treatment among anxious primary care patients. J Nerv Ment Dis 201(3):188–195, 2013 23407203

Hybels CF, Blazer DG: Demography and epidemiology of psychiatric disorders in late life, in The American Psychiatric Publishing Textbook of Geriatric Psychiatry, Fifth Edition. Edited by Steffens DC, Blazer DG, Thakur ME. Washington, DC, American Psychiatric Publishing, 2015, pp 3–32

Institute of Medicine: Unequal Treatment: Confronting Racial and Ethnic Disparities in Health Care. Washington, DC, National Academies Press, 2002

Jimenez DE, Cook B, Bartels SJ, et al: Disparities in mental health service use of racial and ethnic minority elderly adults. J Am Geriatr Soc 61(1):18–25, 2013 23252464

Jones-Webb R: Drinking patterns and problems among African-Americans: recent findings. Alcohol Health Res World 22(4):260–264, 1998 15706752

Joo JH, Wittink M, Dahlberg B: Shared conceptualizations and divergent experiences of counseling among African American and white older adults. Qual Health Res 21(8):1065–1074, 2011 21464469

Kalkonde YV, Pinto-Patarroyo GP, Goldman T, et al: Ethnic disparities in the treatment of dementia in veterans. Dement Geriatr Cogn Disord 28(2):145–152, 2009 19690417

Kasckow J, Ingram E, Brown C, et al: Differences in treatment attitudes between depressed African-American and Caucasian veterans in primary care. Psychiatr Serv 62(4):426–429, 2011 21459996

Klug G, Hermann G, Fuchs-Nieder B, et al: Effectiveness of home treatment for elderly people with depression: randomised controlled trial. Br J Psychiatry 197(6):463–467, 2010 21119152

Komossa K, Rummel-Kluge C, Hunger H, et al: Olanzapine versus other atypical antipsychotics for schizophrenia. Cochrane Database Syst Rev (3):CD006654, 2010 20238348

Krakauer EL, Crenner C, Fox K: Barriers to optimum end-of-life care for minority patients. J Am Geriatr Soc 50(1):182–190, 2002 12028266

Kwak J, Haley WE: Current research findings on end-of-life decision making among racially or ethnically diverse groups. Gerontologist 45(5):634–641, 2005 16199398

Lawson W: Identifying inter-ethnic variations in psychotropic response in African Americans and other ethnic minorities, in Ethnopsychopharmacology. Edited by Ng C, Lin KM, Singh B, et al. Cambridge, UK, Cambridge University Press, 2008, pp 111–117

Lawson WB, Hepler N, Holladay J, Cuffel B: Race as a factor in inpatient and outpatient admissions and diagnosis. Hosp Community Psychiatry 45(1):72–74, 1994 8125467

Lenze EJ, Schultz R, Martire LM, et al: The course of functional decline in older people with persistently elevated depressive symptoms: longitudinal findings from the Cardiovascular Health Study. J Am Geriatr Soc 553(4):569–575, 2005 15817000

Licht-Strunk E, Van Marwijk II, Huekstra T, et al: Outcome of depression in later life in primary care: longitudinal cohort study with three years' follow-up. BMJ 338:a3079, 2009, 19188214

Lester K, Resick PA, Young-Xu Y, et al: Impact of race on early treatment termination and outcomes in posttraumatic stress disorder treatment. J Consult Clin Psychol 78(4):480–489, 2010 20658805

Lilienfeld DE, Perl DP: Projected neurodegenerative disease mortality among minorities in the United States, 1990–2040. Neuroepidemiology 13(4):179–186, 1994 8090260

Lindamer L, Lacro JP, Jeste DV: Relationship of ethnicity to the effects of antipsychotic medication, in Cross Cultural Psychiatry. Edited by Herrara JM, Lawson WB, Stramek JJ. New York, Wiley, 1999, pp 193–203

Luber MP, Meyers BS, Williams-Russo PG, et al: Depression and service utilization in elderly primary care patients. Am J Geriatr Psychiatry 9(2):169–176, 2001 11316621

Lundervold DA, Young LG: Older adults' attitudes and knowledge regarding the use of mental health services. J Clin Exper Gerontology 14:45–55, 1992

Mahoney DF, Cloutterbuck J, Neary S, et al: African American, Chinese, and Latino family caregivers' impressions of the onset and diagnosis of dementia: cross-cultural similarities and differences. Gerontologist 45(6):783–792, 2005 16326660

Marsh JC, Cao D, Guerrero E, et al: Need-service matching in substance abuse treatment: racial/ethnic differences. Eval Program Plann 32(1):43–51, 2009 19019434

Martin SS, Trask J, Peterson T, et al: Influence of culture and discrimination on care-seeking behavior of elderly African Americans: a qualitative study. Soc Work Public Health 25(3):311–326, 2010 20446178

McEvoy JP, Meyer JM, Goff DC, et al: Prevalence of the metabolic syndrome in patients with schizophrenia: baseline results from the Clinical Antipsychotic Trials of Intervention Effectiveness (CATIE) schizophrenia trial and comparison with national estimates from NHANES III. Schizophr Res 80(1):19–32, 2005 16137860

Mechanic D: Mental Health and Social Policy: The Emergence of Managed Care, 4th Edition. Boston, MA, Allyn & Bacon, 1999

Mehta KH, Yin M, Resendez C, et al: Ethnic differences in acetylcholinesterase inhibitor use for Alzheimer disease. Neurology 65(1):159–162, 2005

Meschede T, Sullivan L, Shapiro T: The Crisis of Economic Insecurity for African American and Latino Seniors. New York, Demos, September 2011. Available at: http://www.demos.org/publication/crisis-economic-insecurity-african-american-and-latino-seniors. Accessed May 4, 2018.

Mezuk B, Edwards L, Lohman M, et al: Depression and frailty in later life: a synthetic review. Int J Geriatr Psychiatry 27(9):879–892, 2012 21984056

Miranda J, Duan N, Sherbourne C, et al: Improving care for minorities: can quality improvement interventions improve care and outcomes for depressed minorities? Results of a randomized, controlled trial. Health Serv Res 38(2):613–630, 2003 12785564

Mitchell F: Hoodoo Medicine: Sea Island Herbal Remedies. Berkeley, CA, Reed, Cannon, & Johnson, 1978

Mojtabai R: Increase in antidepressant medication in the US adult population between 1990 and 2003. Psychother Psychosom 77(2):83–92, 2008 18230941

Monroe TB, Carter MA: A retrospective pilot study of African-American and Caucasian nursing home residents with dementia who died from cancer. J Pain Symptom Manage 40(4):e1–e3, 2010 20817471

Mrazek DA, Rush AJ, Biernacka JM, et al: SLC6A4 variation and citalopram response. Am J Med Genet B Neuropsychiatr Genet 150B(3):341–351, 2009 18618621

Mulia N, Ye Y, Greenfield TK, et al: Disparities in alcohol-related problems among white, black, and Hispanic Americans. Alcohol Clin Exp Res 33(4):654–662, 2009 19183131

National Center for Education Statistics: Public High School Graduation Rates. Washington, DC, National Center for Education Statistics, 2017. Available at: https://nces.ed.gov/ccd/tables/ACGR_RF-and_characteristics_2015-16.asp. Accessed May 4, 2018

National Institute of Mental Health: Mental Illness Statistics: Prevalence of Any Mental Illness (AMI). Bethesda, MD, National Institute of Mental Health, 2017. Available at: www.nimh.nih.gov/health/statistics/mental-illness.shtml. Accessed May 4, 2018.

Neighbors HW, Woodward AT, Bullard KM, et al: Mental health service use among older African Americans: the National Survey of American Life. Am J Geriatr Psychiatry 16(12):948–956, 2008 19038893

Niv N, Pham R, Hser YI: Racial and ethnic differences in substance abuse service needs, utilization, and outcomes in California. Psychiatr Serv 60(10):1350–1356, 2009 19797375

Olfson M, Marcus SC, Druss B, et al: National trends in the outpatient treatment of depression. JAMA 287(2):203–209, 2002 11779262

Olfson M, Cherry DK, Lewis-Fernández R: Racial differences in visit duration of outpatient psychiatric visits. Arch Gen Psychiatry 66(2):214–221, 2009 19188544

Omonuwa SC: Health disparity in black women: lack of pharmaceutical advertising in black vs. white-oriented magazines. J Natl Med Assoc 93(7–8):263–266, 2001 11491276

Pickett YR, Weissman J, Bruce ML: Racial differences in antidepressant use among older home health care patients. Psychiatr Serv 63(8):827–829, 2012 22854728

Pickett Y, Bazelias K, Bruce M: Late-life depression in older African Americans: a comprehensive review of epidemiological and clinical data. Int J Geriatr Psychiatry 28(9):903–913, 2013 23225736

Pickett YR, Greenberg RL, Bazelais KN, et al: Depression treatment disparities among older minority home healthcare patients. Am J Geriatr Psychiatry 22(5):519–522, 2014 23711738

Puyat JH, Daw JR, Cunningham CM, et al: Racial and ethnic disparities in the use of antipsychotic medication: a systematic review and meta-analysis. Soc Psychiatry Psychiatr Epidemiol 48(12):1861–1872, 2013 23942793

Quitano LM, Stanley MA, Petersen JM, et al: Healthy IDEAS: a depression intervention delivered by community-based case managers serving older adults. J Appl Gerontol 26:136–156, 2007

Ravenell JE, Johnson WE Jr, Whitaker EE: African-American men's perceptions of health: a focus group study. J Natl Med Assoc 98(4):544–550, 2006 16623067

Richardson TM, Friedman B, Podgorski C, et al: Depression and its correlates among older adults accessing aging services. Am J Geriatr Psychiatry 20(4):346–454, 2012 22434017

Rivers E, Schuman W, Simpson L, et al: Twenty years of follow up experience in long-range medical study. Public Health Rep 68:391–395,1953

Segal SP, Bola JR, Watson MA: Race, quality of care, and antipsychotic prescribing practices in psychiatric emergency services. Psychiatr Serv 47(3):282–286, 1996 8820552

Shellman J, Mokel M, Wright B: Keeping the bully out: understanding older African-Americans perceptions of depression. J Am Psychiatr Nurses Assoc 13:230–236, 2007

Shen H, He MM, Liu H, et al: Comparative metabolic capabilities and inhibitory profiles of CYP2D6.1, CYP2D6.10, and CYP2D6.17. Drug Metab Dispos 35(8):1292–1300, 2007 17470523

Simpson GE: Religious Cults of the Caribbean: Trinidad, Jamaica and Haiti. Rio Piedra, PR, Institute of Caribbean Studies, University of Puerto Rico, 1980

Snowden LR: Barriers to effective mental health services for African Americans. Ment Health Serv Res 3(4):181–187, 2001 11859964

Snowden LR, Pingitore K: Frequency and scope of mental health service delivery to African Americans in primary care. Ment Health Serv Res 4(3):123–130, 2002 12385565

Spector RE: Cultural Diversity in Health and Illness, 9th Edition. Upper Saddle River, NJ, Prentice Hall Health, 2013

Stauffer VL, Sniadecki JL, Piezer KW, et al: Impact of race on efficacy and safety during treatment with olanzapine in schizophrenia, schizophreniform or schizoaffective disorder. BMC Psychiatry 10:89, 2010 21047395

Steffens DC, Fishe G, Langa KM, et al: Prevalence of depression among older Americans: the Aging, Demographics and Memory Study. Int Psychogeriatr 21(5):879–888, 2009 19519984

Stephenson J: Racial barriers may hamper diagnosis, care of patients with Alzheimer disease. JAMA 286(7):779–780, 2001 11497517

Strakowski SM, Keck PE Jr, Arnold LM, et al: Ethnicity and diagnosis in patients with affective disorders. J Clin Psychiatry 64(7):747–754, 2003 12934973

Strickland TL, Lawson W, Lin K, et al: Interethnic variation in response to lithium therapy among African-American and Asian-American populations, in Psychopharmacology and Psychobiology of Ethnicity. Edited by Lin K, Poland RE, Nakasaki G. Washington, DC, American Psychiatric Press, Washington, DC, 1993, pp 107–121

Strickland TL, Lin KM, Fu P, et al: Comparison of lithium ratio between African-American and Caucasian bipolar patients. Biol Psychiatry 37(5):325–330, 1995 7748984

Substance Abuse and Mental Health Services Administration: Results From the 2009 National Survey on Drug Use and Health: Volume I. Summary of National Findings (Office of Applied Studies, NSDUH Series H-38A, HHS Publ No SMA-10-4586). Rockville, MD, Substance Abuse and Mental Health Services Administration, 2010. Available at: www.gmhc.org/files/editor/file/a_pa_nat_drug_use_survey.pdf. Accessed December 23, 2017.

Substance Abuse and Mental Health Services Administration: Results from the 2010 National Survey on Drug Use and Health: Summary of National Findings (Office of Applied Studies, NSDUH Series H-41, HHS Publ No SMA-11-4658). 2011. Available at: https://www.samhsa.gov/data/sites/default/files/NSDUHNationalFindingsResults2010-web/2k10Results-Rev/NSDUHresultsRev2010.pdf. Accessed December 23, 2017.

Tallant R: Voodoo in New Orleans. New York, Collier, 1946

Tang M-X, Cross P, Andrews H, et al: Incidence of AD in African-Americans, Caribbean Hispanics, and Caucasians in northern Manhattan. Neurology 56(1):49–56, 2001 11148235

Taylor RJ, Lincoln KD, Chatters LM: Supportive relationships with church members among African Americans. Fam Relat 54(4):501–511, 2005

Taylor RJ, Chatters LM, Jackson JS: Religious and spiritual involvement among older African Americans, black Caribbeans and whites: findings from the National Survey of American Life. J Gerontol B Psychol Sci Soc Sci 62B:S2, 2007

Tenback DE, van Harten PN, van Os J: Non-therapeutic risk factors for onset of tardive dyskinesia in schizophrenia: a meta-analysis. Mov Disord 24(16):2309–2315, 2009 19645070

Teri L, Gibbons LE, McCurry SM, et al: Exercise plus behavioral management in patients with Alzheimer disease: a randomized controlled trial. JAMA 290(15):2015–2022, 2003 14559955

Thompson VLS, Bazile A, Akbar M: African Americans' perceptions of psychotherapy and psychotherapists. Prof Psychol Res Pr 35:19–26, 2004

Tippett R, Jones-DeWeever A, Rockeymoore M, et al: Beyond Broke: Why Closing the Racial Wealth Gap is a Priority for National Economic Security. Washington, DC, Center for Global Policy Solutions, May 2014. Available at: https://globalpolicysolutions.org/wp-content/uploads/2014/04/BeyondBroke_Exec_Summary.pdf. Accessed May 4, 2018.

Unützer J, Katon W, Callahan CM, et al; IMPACT Investigators. Improving Mood-Promoting Access to Collaborative Treatment: Collaborative care management of late-life depression in the primary care setting: a randomized controlled trial. JAMA 288(22):2836–2845, 2002 12472325

Unützer J, Katon W, Callahan CM, et al: Depression treatment in a sample of 1,801 depressed older adults in primary care. J Am Geriatr Soc 51(4):505–514, 2003 12657070

U.S. Census Bureau: Education, in Statistical Abstract of the United States. Suitland, MD, U.S. Census Bureau, 1999, pp 160–209. Available at: www.census.gov/prod/99pubs/99statab/sec04.pdf. Accessed: May 4, 2018.

U.S. Census Bureau: The Great Migration, 1910 to 1970. Suitland, MD, U.S. Census Bureau, 2012. Available at: www.census.gov/schools/resources/visualizations/great-migration.html. Accessed: May 4, 2018.

U.S. Department of Health and Human Services: Mental Health: Culture, Race, and Ethnicity—A Supplement to Mental Health: A Report of the Surgeon General. Rockville, MD, Center for Mental Health Services, Substance Abuse and Mental Health Services Administration, U.S. Department of Health and Human Services, 2001

Volandes AE, Paasche-Orlow M, Gillick MR, et al: Health literacy not race predicts end-of-life care preferences. J Palliat Med 11(5):754–762, 2008 18588408

Waite KR, Federman AD, McCarthy DM, et al : Literacy and race as risk factors for low rates of advance directives in older adults. J Am Geriatr Soc 61(3):403–406, 2013 23379361

Wang PS, Berglund P, Kessler RC: Recent care of common mental disorders in the United States: prevalence and conformance with evidence-based recommendations. J Gen Intern Med 15(5):284–292, 2000 10840263

Washington H: Medical Apartheid: The Dark History of Medical Experimentation on Black Americans From Colonial Times to the Present. New York, Doubleday, 2007

Waters CM: End-of-life care directives among African Americans: lessons learned—a need for community-centered discussion and education. J Community Health Nurs 17(1):25–37, 2000 10778027

Watson WH: Black Folk Medicine: The Therapeutic Significance of Faith and Trust. New Brunswick, NJ, Transaction Books, 1984

Waxman HM, Carner EA, Klein M: Underutilization of mental health professionals by community elderly. Gerontologist 24(1):23–30, 1984 6698411

West LA, Cole S, Goodkin D, et al: 65+ in the United States: 2010 (Special Studies, Current Population Reports, P23-212). Suitland, MD, U.S. Census Bureau, June 2014. Available at: www.census.gov/content/dam/Census/library/publications/2014/demo/p23-212.pdf. Accessed December 23, 2017.

Wittink MN, Joo JH, Lewis LM, et al: Losing faith and using faith: older African Americans discuss spirituality, religious activities, and depression. J Gen Intern Med 24(3):402–407, 2009 19156471

Woerner MG, Correll CU, Alvir JM, et al: Incidence of tardive dyskinesia with risperidone or olanzapine in the elderly: results from a 2-year, prospective study in antipsychotic-naïve patients. Neuropsychopharmacology 36(8):1738–1746, 2011 21508932

Woodward AT, Taylor RJ, Bullard KM, et al: Prevalence of lifetime DSM-IV affective disorders among older African Americans, black Caribbeans, Latinos, Asians and non-Hispanic white people. Int J Geriatr Psychiatry 27(8):816–827, 2012 21987438

Wu LT, Blazer DG: Illicit and nonmedical drug use among older adults: a review. J Aging Health 23(3):481–504, 2011 21084724

Wulsin LR, Singal BM: Do depressive symptoms increase the risk for the onset of coronary disease? A systematic quantitative review. Psychosom Med 65(2):201–210, 2003 12651987

Yoon Y-H, Yi H-Y, Grant BF, et al: Liver Cirrhosis Mortality in the United States, 1970–98 (Surveillance Rep 57). Bethesda, MD, National Institute on Alcohol Abuse and Alcoholism, December 2001. Available at: https://pubs.niaaa.nih.gov/publications/Cirr98.pdf. Accessed December 23, 2017.

Zaide GB, Pekmezaris R, Nouryan CN, et al: Ethnicity, race, and advance directives in an inpatient palliative care consultation service. Palliat Support Care 11(1):5–11, 2013 22874132

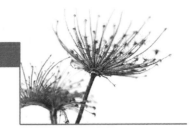

Cultural Competency and Latino Elders

Vicenzio Holder-Perkins, M.D., M.P.H.

Learning Objectives

Develop an understanding of the concepts of culture, ethnicity, race (e.g., Hispanic and black Latinos), nationality, diversity, immigration issues, and acculturation among elderly Latinos residing in the United States.

Develop patient-centered assessments, approaches, and treatment planning in the care of the elderly Latinos that incorporate the diversity and background within their self-described definition of their Latino heritage, including religion, spirituality, and homeopathy.

Learn about elderly Latino groups' shared history of foreign conquest, similar economic and social conditions, and past and present experiences with discrimination and La Migra (Immigration and Naturalization Services).

Develop an approach that destigmatizes mental illnesses among the elderly Latino population and their support system to allow them to trust health care practitioners, receive care and comfort, and access and use the mental health system within the United States regardless of geography.

> Learn about the importance of language in health care de-
> livery and access. Many Latino elderly speak primarily
> Spanish, and their language provides the framework for
> health care practitioners to understand Latino culture,
> which shapes patients' worldview and their health beliefs
> and behaviors.

Definitions clarify the meanings of the terms we use. When precisely formulated and conscientiously followed, definitions make our reasoning more exact and our communication more successful. Unless its meaning is clearly understood, no statement can be empirically verified or logically validated by reference to any other statement. In all scientific fields, but particularly in psychiatry, such clarity of meaning can be achieved only through the most scrupulous efforts to specify these meanings in carefully formulated definitions (Reid and Finesinger 1952).

Culture is defined as the beliefs, customs, language, and history of a similar racial, ethnic, religious, or social community or group. Culture shapes individuals' beliefs, experiences, perceptions, and decisions and how the individual relates to others. It influences the way patients respond to medical recommendations and treatment, social services, and preventive interventions and can also have an impact on the way clinicians or health care professionals deliver those services.

Cultural competence is a set of congruent behaviors, attitudes, and policies that facilitate a professional, a practice, or an agency coming together as a system to work effectively in cross-cultural situations. The word *culture* implies an integrated pattern of human thoughts, communications, actions, customs, beliefs, values, and institutions of a racial, ethnic, religious, or social group. *Competence* indicates having the capacity and expertise to function effectively (Cohen and Goode 1999). Professional competence requires that the clinician practice in a manner that considers each patient's cultural and linguistic characteristics and unique values so that the most effective assessment and intervention services can be provided.

DEFINITIONS OF THE TERMS LATINO
AND HISPANIC

One may wonder about the choice of the term Latino and not Hispanic for this title of chapter. *Hispanic* refers to language and is used to denote the culture and people of countries formerly ruled by the Spanish Empire, where the majority of the population usually speaks the Spanish language. In the United States, the term was first adopted during the administration of Richard Nixon and has been used for the U.S. Census since 1980. *Latino*, on the other hand, refers to a geographic region. People who live in the Caribbean (e.g., Puerto Rico, Cuba, Dominican Republic), South America (e.g., Ecuador, Bolivia, Colombia, Peru) and Central America (e.g., Panama, Honduras, Costa Rica) are from Latin America and are referred to as Latin Americans.

The U.S. government adopted the word Latino as an inclusive term to refer to people from all races who are of Latin American nationality and their U.S.-born descendants who live in the United States. These individuals speak primarily Romance languages (Spanish or Portuguese), although Native American languages are also spoken by some. Researchers and federal data sources also often use the terms *Spanish origin*, *Spanish speaking*, and *Spanish surnamed* synonymously for Latinos. These terms unfortunately suffer from the same limitations as Hispanic in identifying and classifying individuals for the purposes of research and planning (Lopez 2014; Valdez and Arce 2000).

The 2006 Latino National Survey (Fraga et al. 2013) found that 35% of respondents preferred the term Hispanic, whereas 13.4% preferred the term Latino. More than 32% of respondents reported that either term was acceptable, and 18.1% indicated they did not care. In this chapter, because of the variable use of *Hispanic* and *Latino* in the literature, research, and publications, these terms will be used interchangeably to refer to peoples of Latin American origin living in the United States.

Origin can be seen as the heritage, nationality group, lineage, or country of birth of the person or the person's parents or ancestors prior to arrival in the United States. People who identify their origin as Spanish, Hispanic, or Latino may be of any race or mixed race.

CENSUS DEMOGRAPHICS OF
U.S. LATINO ELDERLY

In 2014, there were 46.2 million Americans age 65 years and older and 6.2 million age 85 years and older (Adminstration for Community Living 2015a). All Americans are living longer, and the same is true for the Hispanic population. The Hispanic older population (of any race) numbered 3.6 million in 2014 and is projected to grow to 21.5 million by 2060. In 2014, Hispanics made up 8% of the older population. By 2060, the percentage of the older population that is Hispanic is projected to be 22%.

The three largest subgroups of Hispanics in the United States come from Mexico, Puerto Rico, and Cuba, and more than half of Latino elders age 60 and older are of Mexican heritage. Almost all Cuban, Central American, and South American elders in the United States are currently foreign born. Hispanics live longer than whites. According to the *National Vital Statistic Reports*, overall, 87.2% of the Hispanic population survived to age 65, compared with 84.3% of the non-Hispanic white and 74.7% of the non-Hispanic black populations (Arias 2012). The Hispanic survival advantage increases with age so that by age 85 nearly one-half (48.9%) of the Hispanic population has survived, compared with 40.0% of the non-Hispanic white and 29.9% of the non-Hispanic black populations. In 2014, there were 5,272 Hispanics age 100 years and older (1,397 men and 3,875 women), comprising 7% of all centenarians (Administration for Community Living 2015b). As Latino life expectancy increases and the net levels of immigration increase, the number of elderly Latinos could be even higher.

PORTRAIT OF U.S. ELDERLY LATINOS

Although Latino elders are a heterogeneous group, almost all share the Spanish language, albeit with regional variations. However, some Latino elders do not speak Spanish at all; for example, some Indigenous elders who have emigrated from Mexico speak only Nahuatl (known historically as Aztec), a language or group of languages of the Uto-Aztecan language family. The majority of these Nahuatl speakers migrated from central Mexico, particularly Puebla, Veracruz, Hidalgo, San Luis Potosí, Guerrero, México (state), El Distrito Federal, Tlaxcala, Morelos, and Oaxaca. Most Mexican-origin elderly Latinos live in the western United States, primarily in California. A significant number of this population also live in the Southwest, particularly in Texas (Horizons Project 2000).

Latinos, regardless of age, also share numerous common backgrounds and circumstances. For example, Latinos have comparable origins in tribal societies and a history of foreign conquest, colonialism, and neocolonialism. Colonial expansion under the crown of Castile was initiated by the Spanish conquistadores and was developed by its administrators and missionaries. The motivations for colonial expansion were trade and the spread of the Catholic faith through Indigenous conversions. Beginning with the 1492 arrival of Christopher Columbus and continuing for more than three centuries, the Spanish Empire expanded across the Caribbean Islands, half of South America, most of Central America, and much of North America, including present-day Mexico, Florida, and the Southwest and Pacific Coastal regions of the United States. It is estimated that during the colonial period (1492–1832), a total of 18.6 million Spaniards settled in the Americas, and a further 3.5 million immigrated during the postcolonial era (1850–1950). In the early nineteenth century, a series of Spanish-American wars of independence resulted in the emancipation of most of the Spanish colonies in the Americas. Cuba and Puerto Rico, together with Guam and the Philippines in the Pacific, were finally given up in 1898 following the Spanish-American War. Spain's loss of these last territories politically ended Spanish rule in the Americas (Gonzalez-Barrera and Lopez 2013).

Latinos comprise a mosaic group who share similar economic and social conditions and have past and present experiences with discrimination and health care disparities. The Centers for Disease Control and Prevention define health disparities as "preventable differences, in the burden of disease, injury, violence, or opportunities to achieve optimal health that are experienced by socially disadvantaged populations" such as elderly Latinos (Centers for Disease Control and Prevention 2011, p. 3).

Communication barriers within the elderly Latino community cause numerous disparities that are currently being experienced by this population. Most elderly Latino migrants speak Spanish as their primary or native language and once situated in a predominantly Latino community have no need to learn English. Their personal needs are met by immediate family at home or by the Latino community at large. Language is as much about value, culture, identity, context, emotion, behavior, and usage. It provides a frame of reference in which an individual's worldview is shaped, including health beliefs and behaviors.

Health care, however, often requires some ability to read or speak English. Over the past several decades, several published surveys and studies have found the existence of health disparities due to communication barriers. Half or more of Spanish speakers reported problems communicating with or understanding their health care provider (Schur and Albers 1996). Among Latinos, studies indicate that Spanish speakers are less likely than English speakers to have a usual source of health care (Schur and Albers 1996). In an evaluation of the Consumer Assessment of Healthcare Providers and Systems health plan surveys, Hispanics who spoke Spanish reported worse experiences than whites regarding timeliness of care provider communication, staff helpfulness, and health plan service (Morales et al. 2001). Productive interactions with health care providers lead to a sense that the patient has been respected and listened to and facilitate the achievement of optimal health outcomes for the elderly Latino.

CULTURE AND HEALTH

Latinos come from a collectivistic culture where group activities are dominant, responsibility is shared, and accountability is collective. This leads to an emphasis on the group more than individual function and responsibility. Most Latinos or Hispanics believe that God is an active force in everyday life. Most pray every day, have a religious object in their home, and attend religious services. Faith and church are often central to family and community life and are important in the understanding of illness and healing.

The meaning of *health* varies among Latinos. Some maintain that health results from good luck or is a reward for good behavior. Illnesses may have either natural or supernatural causes. Symptoms are often interpreted differently on the basis of cultural presuppositions. Non-Latino health care providers, including mental health providers, may be perplexed by references to folk healing and illness in Latino patients regardless of age.

Latino healing traditions include *curanderismo* in Mexico and much of Latin America, *Santería* in Brazil and Cuba, and *espiritismo* in Puerto Rico (Spector 2004). *Curanderos,* traditional healers, distinguish between "hot" and "cold" illnesses and occasionally between natural and unnatural (sorcery-related) diseases (Zoucha et al. 2003). Latinos may seek out the care of *brujos* (wizards) or *brujas* (witches) for the latter conditions. Other healing specialists include *yerberas* (herbalists), *hueseros* (bonesetters), *parteras* (midwives), and *sobradores* (similar to physical therapists) (Fernandez 1998).

Clinicians need to consider the effects of culture when diagnosing psychiatric conditions. DSM-5 makes it clear that understanding the cultural context of illness experience is essential for effective diagnostic assessment and clinical management (American Psychiatric Association 2013). The Center for Substance Abuse Treatment (2014) provides a systematic outline for incorporating culturally relevant information. Clinicians can use the main content areas listed below to guide the interview, initial intake, and treatment planning processes. For immigrants and ethnic minorities, one should note the degree of involvement with culture of origin and host culture (where applicable). Language ability, use, and preference (including multilingualism) also should be evaluated. DSM-5 suggests an outline for cultural formulation that calls for systematic assessment of the following categories:

1. Cultural identity of the individual
2. Cultural conceptualizations of distress (Table 7–1)

3. Psychosocial stressors and cultural features of vulnerability and resilience
4. Cultural features of the relationship between the individual and the clinician
5. Overall cultural assessment

TABLE 7–1. Latino cultural concepts of distress

Name	Description
Mal puesto (sorcery)	Unnatural illness that is not easily explained.
Pasmo ("frozen face")	Temporary paralysis of the face or limbs, often thought to be caused by a sudden hot-cold imbalance.
Susto ("soul loss")	Posttraumatic illness (e.g., shock, insomnia, depression, anxiety).
Ataque de nervios	Out-of-consciousness state resulting from evil spirits. Symptoms include attacks of crying, trembling, uncontrollable shouting, physical or verbal aggression, and intense heat in the chest moving to the head. These events are often associated with stressful events (e.g., death of a loved one, witnessing an accident involving a family member).
Cólera	Anger and rage disturbing body balances and leading to headache, screaming, stomach pain, loss of consciousness, and fatigue.
Mal de ojo ("evil eye")	Medical problems such as GI symptoms, anxiety, and depression could result from *mal de ojo* the individual experienced from another person. It is common among infants and children; adults might also experience it.
Wind or cold illness	Anxiety or fear of cold and the wind; feeling weakness and susceptibility to illness resulting from the belief that natural and supernatural elements are not balanced.

Note. GI=gastrointestinal.

Cultural Normative Values and Approaches to Treatment

Latino culture has several normative values that should be recognized in clinical settings. These include *simpatía* (kindness), *personalismo* (friendliness), and *respeto* (respect) (Flores et al. 2000). *Simpatía* emphasizes politeness and conflict avoidance. *Personalismo*, a personal connection, can be achieved by asking about the patient and his or her family. Because people stand closer to each other in most Latino cultures than is typical in American culture, physical proximity is also perceived as being more personable. *Respeto* implies attentive concern for the patient and respect of his or her personhood and age, especially if the patient is older. Older patients should be addressed as *señor* or *señora* rather than by their first names. Using *don* or *doña* with the given or full name indicates even greater respect for older patients.

Addressing patients properly can be a challenge. Double or hyphenated Latino surnames may seem complicated, with the father's name preceding the mother's. Additionally, when a woman gets married, her husband's name may be appended to her father's name. Some Latinos adopt American naming conventions, but others do not. When in doubt, the best policy is to ask the patient how he or she would like to be addressed (Galanti 2008).

Additionally, the cultural value of *modestia* (modesty), which is related to respect, is often unrecognized (Juckett 2013). Latinos may be conservative in this area, and physical exposure should be negotiated as the examination warrants. A chaperone is often appreciated if a same-sex physician is not available.

Although patients of all cultural backgrounds warrant kindness, a personal connection, and respect, the consequences of failing to include these traditional values may be more problematic with Latinos. In Latino cultures, the elderly are believed to have inner strength. Latino elderly occupy a central role in the family and are treated with *respeto*, acknowledging their status (i.e., their place within the family) and authority, which derives from years of life experiences.

Frequent visits by their children play a major role in caring for aging Latinos and providing assistance. The assistance by their children is expected and does not result in diminished feelings of self-worth. This cultural norm among the elderly Latino has an impact on Hispanic family members who are in the role of caregivers and poses challenges for non-Hispanics who may be surprised when families resist the recommendation to institutionalize an older member of the family, especially a parent.

Providers working with Latinos also may need to understand how to target health messages differently to older men and women. Understanding these concepts can facilitate the negotiation of family dynamics. Latinos typically subscribe to values of *machismo* and *marianismo* that culturally define the male and female roles. There are Latino men who hold the value of *machismo* to be so true that they are often reluctant to seek medical care until they are so sick that a visit to an emergency department is required. In addition, the Latino male figure may take a controversial stance on the health care needs of family members (Parangimalil 2001).

Marianismo is an aspect of the female gender role in the machismo of Hispanic American folk culture. It is the veneration for feminine virtues such as purity and "moral" strength. Female gender roles have been linked to a number of negative health outcomes in populations across the United States. For instance, various studies have demonstrated a strong link between experiences of sexism and gender inequality and rates of psychological distress, including symptoms of depression and anxiety (e.g., Fischer and Holz 2007; Klono et al. 2000; Moradi et al. 2006). Specifically, the adherence to strict, traditional gender roles has been shown to play a role in symptomology among women (Sweeting et al. 2014). Sweeting et al. (2014) also found that as gender roles and gender role beliefs become more egalitarian between males and females, the excessive prevalence of major depressive disorder in females decreases.

Terms for psychiatric illness also have unique meanings. Mental disorder (*enfermedad mental, crisis*, or *ataque de nervios*) is a less stigmatized term than being "insane" (*estar loco*). *Nervios* is a culturally acceptable and nonstigmatizing term for emotional or psychological distress and illness among Latinos. If a person is *loco*, then he or she has a complete loss of control or withdrawal, or *locura*. *Locura* is a term used by Latinos in the United States and Latin America to refer to a severe form of psychiatric illness, typically of a psychotic nature. The condition is attributed to an inherited vulnerability, to the effect of multiple life difficulties, or to a combination of both factors. Symptoms exhibited by persons with *locura* include incoherence, agitation, auditory and visual hallucinations, an inability to follow normed rules of social interaction, unpredictability, and possibly violence.

Elderly Latinos, not unlike members of other ethnic cultures, are known to use herbal medicines. These herbs may include spearmint, chamomile, aloe vera, garlic, brook mint, osha lavender, ginger, and oregano, to name a few (Zeilmann et al. 2003). It is also not unusual for Latinos to find medicinal powers in fruit such as papaya, pineapple, and citrus fruits. Providers should inquire as to the use of these naturo-pathics, which are often consumed as herbal teas.

Acculturation and Assimilation

The aforementioned Latino cultural normative values, as they relate to patients' approach to care and perception of mental illness, are distinct from acculturation and assimilation, which are terms used to describe the complex processes that immigrants go through as they incorporate into a host society's culture. *Acculturation* is a process of cultural contact and exchange through which people or groups come to adopt certain values and practices of a culture that is not originally their own, to a greater or lesser extent. The end result is that the original culture of the person or group remains but is changed by this process. *Assimilation* is used when little to no importance is placed on maintaining the original culture and great importance is put on fitting in and developing rela-tionships with the new culture. The outcome is that the person or group is, eventually, culturally indistinguishable from the culture into which they have assimilated. This type of acculturation is likely to occur in so-cieties that are considered to "melting pots" into which new members are absorbed.

Acculturation and assimilation include a range of contextual and in-dividual-level factors that interact in ways unique to each immigrant. Hence, a "one-size-fits-all" approach for access to and provision of mental health services is inadequate for Latino immigrants. Latino newcomers to the United States vary in many aspects, including their demographics, life experiences in their countries of origin, and reasons for migration. At the same time, the sociopolitical climate of the United States constantly changes, making it nearly impossible to predict how the current wave of Latino immigrants will acculturate. Such is the case with Latino elders, who have different levels of acculturation and as-similation. Unlike some other immigrant groups, many Latinos in the United States, regardless of the region in which they reside (e.g., the Los Angeles, Chicago, Greater New York, and Miami metropolitan areas and the states of Nevada, Arizona, New Mexico, and Colorado), retain the traditions and health behaviors of their native countries.

As theories of acculturation have evolved and informed our under-standing of the immigrant experience, our appreciation of the psycho-logical stressors that surround this transition has deepened. It is not surprising that many of the issues that bring Latino immigrants to men-tal health systems stem from tensions caused by acculturation pro-cesses. Unfortunately, the effects of acculturation on the mental health of Latinos are not well understood (Lopez 2014). All in all, behavioral changes occurring during acculturation do not occur uniformly for all individuals. Rather, it is believed that acculturation occurs in each person in different ways and at different rates. During the course of the acculturation process, the many contextual interactions in which immigrants' lives are embedded have significant and multifaceted effects on emotional experiences.

MENTAL ILLNESS AND ELDERLY LATINOS IN THE UNITED STATES

The U.S. Department of Health and Human Services Office of Minority Health has written about difficulties of health care access for at-risk populations such as elderly Latinos (Agency for Healthcare Research and Quality 2014). These researchers have calculated the occurrence rates of stress-related illnesses and psychological symptoms. Wherever a significantly higher rate of an illness or symptom occurs in the Latino immigrant sample compared with Latino American or white American prevalence rates, the authors underline a cause for concern and discuss concentrated effects.

Acculturation is inherently stressful because individuals must come to terms with different cultural norms, some of which conflict with those of their country of origin. Mental health ultimately depends on how successfully the individual is able to cope with the stressors encountered. Person-level resources, including coping mechanisms, social supports, and adequate skills, greatly influence acculturation outcomes. Latinos may believe that family issues, migration, and the loss of family and friends cause mental disorders (Kramer et al. 2009). Among psychiatric disorders, adjustment disorder is highly prevalent among immigrant Latinos and may be due to the effects and impact of acculturation to the culture of the United States. Additionally, higher levels of acculturation are positively correlated with higher odds of alcohol consumption among Latino women, but this relationship is weaker among men (Zemore 2007).

Lower rates of depression as well as better physical functioning have been reported among Hispanic immigrants compared with U.S.-born Latinos (Escobar et al. 2000). Most of these studies were in the Mexican subgroup. Other studies, however, have found higher rates of depression symptoms among Latino elderly (González et al. 2001), which varied as much as twofold on the basis of Hispanic background

(Puerto Rican and Cuban) and gender as well as history of and risk factors for cardiovascular disease (Wassertheil-Smoller et al. 2014). Antidepressant medication use among Latinos was lower than in the general population, suggesting undertreatment. Among Mexican Americans, studies have found that place of birth is strongly correlated with incidence of mental illness. Individuals born in Mexico exhibit lower incidence and prevalence of mental illness compared with U.S.-born Mexican Americans (Vega et al. 1998). This difference disappears the longer the person lives in the United States, such that once 13 years have passed, incidence rates approach that of the non-Hispanic American population.

In a report issued in 2014 by the U.S. Department of Health and Human Services Office of Minority Health (Agency for Healthcare Research and Quality 2014), the suicide rates for Latino men older than age 65 was 15.9, compared with 36.1 for non-Latino white men. Suicide rates for Latino women older than age 65 was 2.1, versus 5.8 for non-Latino white women. In general, suicide rates among Latino elderly immigrants were low, with one exception: Cuba has higher rates of suicide than other countries in the Americas, and older Cuban men living in the United States have been found to have suicide rates that were 1.67 times higher than those of their non-Hispanic counterparts (Llorente et al. 1996).

A growing body of evidence suggests that Alzheimer's disease may disproportionately affect minority groups in the United States. After adjusting for gender and comorbidities, Hispanics have a statistically higher risk than non-Hispanic whites for developing Alzheimer's disease (Chen and Panegyres 2016). In a 7-year community-based study, Tang et al. (2001) sampled and interviewed Medicare recipients age 65 years and older in New York City. They found that the cumulative incidence of Alzheimer's disease ages 65–90 years was approximately two times greater in Caribbean Hispanic individuals than among white non-Hispanic individuals. These analyses controlled for medical history, such as history of heart disease, stroke, and cardiovascular and cerebrovascular disorders, as well as other demographic factors, such as level of education and literacy. Nevertheless, the lack of a population-based sample in these studies hinders the generalization of these results (Chen and Panegyres 2016; Chin et al. 2011).

MENTAL HEALTH SERVICES

Mental health providers in the United States encounter challenges when engaging with the rapidly growing population of Hispanic older adults in evidence-based mental health treatments. This population underutilizes mental health services, despite comparable or slightly higher rates of mental illness compared with non-Hispanic white older adults (Derr 2016). Results of a study of disparities in mental health service use showed that treatment initiation and adequacy were lower for older Latinos than they were for older non-Latino whites (Horizons Project 2000). These disparities persist even after adjusting for severity of mental and physical health conditions, demographic characteristics (e.g., socioeconomic status, education level), and insurance coverage.

Stigma and lack of understanding regarding mental disorders and their treatments may play a role in lower utilization of mental health services. Several characteristics have been linked with this stigma among Latinos regardless of age (Kramer et al. 2009) and include the following:

- Negative cultural undertones associated with mental illness—In many Latino cultures, mental disorders are highly stigmatized. Having a mental disorder is viewed as a sign of personal weakness. As a result, distress is more likely to be verbalized using somatic terms and symptoms rather than psychiatric symptoms. For example, an older Latino adult may report vague somatic symptoms and *nervios* rather than psychological distress.
- Stress of immigration and acculturation experiences—Traditional Latino cultures value family cohesion within well-structured roles. Migration often upsets these roles. Migration can separate families and strain relationships. Over time, marriages may break up. Relatives who provide support may be left behind, and family dynamics may change as children acculturate more quickly than their parents. For many migrants, the stress of relocation heightens as they encounter American society, with its emphasis on individual independence from the nuclear or extended family. This stress is further heightened through the experiences of discrimination from the wider community.

The stigma of having a mental illness is one of the most significant obstacles preventing Latinos from seeking mental health services. Immigration status is likely another deterrent to mental health care utilization in the United States. Lack of access to mental health services and low utilization of these services have been found to be more pronounced among men and the uninsured, with the lowest utilization rates among undocumented Latino immigrants (Kedem 2015).

Providing outreach to older adults and engaging them in services to prevent and address psychiatric illness and substance abuse can be challenging. The high prevalence of certain mental disorders, low use of mental health services, differing beliefs about mental health issues, and the stigma associated with mental illness illustrate the need to create culturally appropriate interventions for older racial and ethnic minorities.

Conclusion

Hispanics living in the United States represent a highly diverse group of individuals from several countries. Relatively new groups, including Dominicans, Salvadorans, Guatemalans, and Colombians, have grown rapidly, adding their numbers to well-established populations of Mexican, Puerto Rican, and Cuban origin (Horizons Project 2000).

As the United States ages over the next several decades, its older population will become more racially and ethnically diverse. Latinos are the largest ethnic minority group in the United States. With a population of approximately 45 million, they now constitute 14% of the total U.S. population. By 2050, because of population growth through migration and higher birth rates, Latinos will account for 25% of the U.S. population (Centers for Disease Control and Prevention 2015). This projected growth will present challenges to policy makers and to programs such as Social Security and Medicare. It will also affect businesses and health care providers. The Centers for Disease Control and Prevention (2015) recommend that all health care providers play a key role in helping to provide culturally and linguistically appropriate outreach to Latino patients and reinforce the need to sustain strong community, public health, and health care linkages that support Hispanic health. Cultural insights and competency are imperative in engaging the Latino patient in a health care setting.

Knowledge of the central role that culture plays allows for appropriate utilization of health care services and better health care outcomes. When conducting mental and/or physical assessments, providers must always keep in the forefront the knowledge that there is cultural diversity within the Latino population. Latinos are highly diverse and consist of subgroups, such as Mexicans, Cubans, Puerto Ricans, Panamanians, Dominicans, and Salvadorans, who differ in their migration experiences and reasons for migrating, lifestyles, health beliefs, and health practices. Professional competence requires that the clinician practice in a manner that considers each person's cultural and linguistic characteristics and unique values so that the most effective assessment and intervention services can be provided (Centers for Disease Control and Prevention 2015).

KEY POINTS

- The Latino population is extremely diverse across a number of dimensions, including country of origin, immigration status, language use, ethnic and racial background, religious and spiritual beliefs, and generation in the United States.
- In addition to culture-bound syndromes unique to Latino elders, all psychiatric conditions can be found in Latino groups, although there may be variants of clinical presentations, as well as in how Latinos interpret treatment recommendations.
- Stigma associated with mental health conditions and treatment is a significant barrier to access to care and must be overcome.
- Certain mental health conditions are more prevalent among Latino elderly, in particular Alzheimer's disease.
- Immigration, adaptation, and acculturation play important roles in the prevalence and incidence of psychiatric disorders among older Latinos.

QUESTIONS FOR FURTHER THOUGHT

1. True or False: Latino elders are a homogeneous group, and the one and only common thread is that they speak Spanish.

2. Latino culture has three normative values that must be recognized in any clinical setting. List these values.

3. True or False: Suicide rates among all Latino elderly immigrants are generally low.

4. Strategies for creating a culturally sensitive environment for Latino patients include which of the following?

    A. Allowing extra time for patients with limited English proficiency.
    B. Posting bilingual or Spanish language signage.
    C. Providing culturally sensitive training for staff.
    D. All of the above.

SUGGESTED READINGS AND WEBSITES

Butterfield, S: Consider country, culture when caring for Latino populations. Presented at the American College of Physicians Internal Medicine Meeting, Orlando, FL, June 2014. Available at: https://acpinternist.org/archives/2014/06/cultural.htm.

Centers for Disease Control and Prevention: Cultural Insights: Communicating With Hispanics/Latinos. Atlanta, GA, Centers for Disease Control and Prevention, 2017. Available at: www.cdc.gov/healthcommunication/pdf/audience/audienceinsight_cultural insights.pdf.

Evercare and National Alliance for Caregiving: Evercare Study of Hispanic Family Caregiving in the U.S. Bethesda, MD, National Alliance for Caregiving, 2008. Available at: www.caregiving.org/data/Hispanic_Caregiver_Study_web_ENG_FINAL_11_04_08.pdf.

REFERENCES

Administration for Community Living: A Statistical Profile of Older Americans. Washington, DC, Administration for Community Living, 2015a. Available at: www.acl.gov/sites/default/files/news%202017-03/A_Statistical_Profile_of_Older_Americans.pdf. Accessed May 7, 2018.

Administration for Community Living: Statistical Profile of Older Hispanic Americans. Washington, DC, Administration for Community Living, 2015b. Available at: www.acl.gov/sites/default/files/Aging%20and%20Disability%20in%20America/Statistical-Profile-Older-Hispanic-Ameri.pdf. Accessed May 7, 2018.

Agency for Healthcare Research and Quality: National Healthcare Quality and Disparities Reports. Data Query: Table 6_7_1_1_1.1. Rockville, MD, Office of Minority Health, 2014. Available at: http://nhqrnet.ahrq.gov/inhqrdr/data/query. Accessed June 20, 2016.

American Psychiatric Association: Diagnostic and Statistical Manual of Mental Disorders, 5th Edition, Arlington, VA, American Psychiatric Association, 2013

Arias E: United States Life Tables 2008 (National Vital Statistics Rep Vol 61, No 3). Hyattsville, MD, National Center for Health Statistics, September 24, 2012. Available at: www.cdc.gov/nchs/data/nvsr/nvsr61/nvsr61_03.pdf. Accessed May 29, 2018.

Center for Substance Abuse Treatment: Improving Cultural Competence (TIP 59, Report No SMA 14-4849). Rockville, MD, Substance Abuse and Mental Health Services Administration, 2014

Centers for Disease Control and Prevention: CDC Health Disparities and Inequalities Report—United States, 2011. MMWR Suppl Vol 60. Atlanta, GA, Centers for Disease Control and Prevention, January 14 2011. Available at: www.cdc.gov/mmwr/pdf/other/su6001.pdf. Accessed December 28, 2017.

Centers for Disease Control and Prevention: Hispanics' Health in the United States. Atlanta, GA, Centers for Disease Control and Prevention, May 5, 2015. Available at: www.cdc.gov/media/releases/2015/p0505-hispanic-health.html. Accessed December 28, 2017.

Chen HY, Panegyres PK: The role of ethnicity in Alzheimer's disease: findings from the C-PATH online data repository. J Alzheimers Dis 51(2):515–523, 2016 26890783

Chin AL, Negash S, Hamilton R: Diversity and disparity in dementia: the impact of ethnoracial differences in Alzheimer disease. Alzheimer Dis Assoc Disord 25(3):187–195, 2011 21399486

Cohen E, Goode TD: Policy Brief 1: Rationale for Cultural Competence in Primary Health Care. Washington, DC, National Center for Cultural Competence, 1999

Derr AS: Mental health service use among immigrants in the United States: a systematic review. Psychiatr Serv 67(3):265–274, 2016 26695493

Escobar JI, Hoyos Nervi C, Gara MA: Immigration and mental health: Mexican Americans in the United States. Harv Rev Psychiatry 8(2):64–72, 2000 10902095

Fernandez C: Discovering curanderismo, in Healing Latinos: Realidad y Fantasia: The Art of Cultural Competence in Medicine. Edited by Hayes-Bautista DE. Los Angeles, CA, Center for the Study of Latino Health/UCLA, 1998, pp 187–202

Fischer AR, Holz KB: Perceived discrimination and women's psychological distress: the roles of collective and personal self-esteem. J Couns Psychol 54:154–164, 2007

Flores G, Abreu M, Schwartz I, et al: The importance of language and culture in pediatric care: case studies from the Latino community. J Pediatr 137(6):842–848, 2000 11113842

Fraga LR, Garcia JA, Hero R, et al: Latino National Survey (LNS), 2006 (ICPSR 20862). Ann Arbor, MI, Inter-university Consortium for Political and Social Research, 2013

Galanti G: Communication and time orientation, in Caring for Patients From Different Cultures, 4th Edition. Philadelphia, University of Pennsylvania Press, 2008, pp 27–51

González HM, Haan MN, Hinton L: Acculturation and the prevalence of depression in older Mexican Americans: baseline results of the Sacramento Area Latino Study on Aging. J Am Geriatr Soc 49(7):948–953, 2001 11527487

Gonzalez-Barrera A, Lopez HA: A Demographic Portrait of Mexican-Origin Hispanics in the United States. Washington, DC, Pew Research Center, May 1, 2013. Available at: www.pewhispanic.org/2013/05/01/a-demographic-portrait-of-mexican-origin-hispanics-in-the-united-states. Accessed December 28, 2017.

Horizons Project: Nationwide Demographic Report, Final (Contract 500-99-0036). San Antonio, TX, Cutting Edge Communications, NuStats International, 2000

Juckett G: Caring for Latino patients. Am Fam Physician 87(1):48–54, 2013 23317025

Kedem S: Associative factors of acculturative stress in Latino immigrants. Doctoral dissertation, Walden University, 2015, pp 3–17

Klono EA, Landrine H, Campbell R: Sexist discrimination may account for well-known gender differences in psychiatric symptoms. Psychol Women Q 24:93–99, 2000

Kramer EJ, Guarnaccia P, Resendez C, et al: ¡No Soy Loco!/I'm not Crazy! Understanding the Stigma of Mental Illness in Latinos (video). Seattle, WA Ethnomed, January 1, 2009. Available at: https://ethnomed.org/clinical/mental-health/NoSoyLoco.flv/view. Accessed January 2, 2018.

Lopez RA: Latino Opinion: A Collection of Latino Opinions. New York, Hispanic Research, 2014. Available at: www.latinoopinion.com. Accessed January 2, 2018.

Llorente MD, Eisdorfer C, Zarate Y, et al: Suicide among Hispanic elderly: Cuban-Americans in Dade County, Florida, 1990–93. J Ment Health Aging (2):79–87, 1996

Moradi B, Funderburk JR: Roles of perceived sexist events and perceived social support in the mental health of women seeking counseling. J Couns Psychol 53:464–473, 2006

Morales LS, Elliott MN, Weech-Maldonado R, et al: Differences in CAHPS adult survey reports and ratings by race and ethnicity: an analysis of the National CAHPS benchmarking data 1.0. Health Serv Res 36(3):595–617, 2001 11482591

Parangimalil GJ: Latino health in the new millennium: the need for a culture-centered approach. Sociol Spectr 21(3):423–429, 2001

Reid JR, Finesinger JE: The role of definitions in psychiatry. Am J Psychiatry 109(6):413–420, 1952 12986007

Schur CL, Albers LA: Language, sociodemographics, and health care use of Hispanic adults. J Health Care Poor Underserved 7(2):140–158, 1996 8935388

Spector RE: Health and illness in Hispanic Americans, in Cultural Diversity in Health and Illness, 6th Edition. Upper Saddle River, NJ, Pearson Prentice Hall, 2004, pp 253–278

Sweeting H, Bhaskar A, Benzeval M, et al: Changing gender roles and attitudes and their implications for well-being around the new millennium. Soc Psychiatry Psychiatr Epidemiol 49(5):791–809, 2014 23907414

Tang MX, Cross P, Andrews H, et al: Incidence of AD in African-Americans, Caribbean Hispanics, and Caucasians in northern Manhattan. Neurology 56(1):49–56, 2001 11148235

Valdez RB, Arce C: A Profile of Hispanic Elders. Baltimore, MD, Horizons Project, Health Care Financing Administration, 2000. Available at: http://latino.si.edu/virtualgallery/growingold/Nationwide%20Demographic.pdf. Accessed January 2, 2018.

Vega WA, Kolody B, Aguilar-Gaxiola S, et al: Lifetime prevalence of DSM-III-R psychiatric disorders among urban and rural Mexican Americans in California. Arch Gen Psychiatry 55(9):771–778, 1998 9736002

Wassertheil-Smoller S, Arredondo EM, Cai J, et al: Depression, anxiety, antide-
    pressant use, and cardiovascular disease among Hispanic men and women
    of different national backgrounds: results from the Hispanic Community
    Health Study/Study of Latinos. Ann Epidemiol 24(11):822–830, 2014
    25439033
Zeilmann CA, Dole EJ, Skipper BJ, et al: Use of herbal medicine by elderly His-
    panic and non-Hispanic white patients. Pharmacotherapy 23(4):526–532,
    2003 12680482
Zemore SE: Acculturation and alcohol among Latino adults in the United
    States: a comprehensive review. Alcohol Clin Exp Res 31(12):1968–1990,
    2007 18034692
Zoucha R, Purnell LD: People of Mexican heritage, in Transcultural Health
    Care: A Culturally Competent Approach, 2nd Edition. Edited by Purnell
    LD, Paulanka BJ. Philadelphia, PA, F A Davis, 2003, pp 264–278

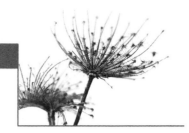

CHAPTER 8

Older Lesbian, Gay, Bisexual, and Transgender Adults

R. Dakota Carter, M.D.
Siddarth Puri, M.D.
Rebecca Radue, M.D.
Daniel D. Sewell, M.D.

Learning Objectives

Appreciate the general size of the older lesbian, gay, bisexual, and transgender (LGBT) population in the United States.

Recognize the diversity that exists within the LGBT community and understand the term *intersectionality* and how it applies to older members of the LGBT community.

Learn and use properly various terms necessary for providing optimal health care to older members of the LGBT community.

Become familiar with the health disparities currently observed in the LGBT community.

Provide examples of how the aging process may uniquely impact older members of the LGBT community.

List a number of steps that providers can take to ensure that their practice environments are welcoming and inclusive to members of the LGBT community.

There are between 2.7 and 4 million lesbian, gay, bisexual, or transgender (LGBT) individuals older than age 50 years in the United States, with 1.1 million LGBT individuals older than age 65 years, according to the LGBT+ National Aging Research Center (Fredriksen-Goldsen and Muraco 2010). Given that by 2030 as much as 20% of the population will be 65 years old or older, the number of older LGBT community members in the United States may reach 6 million (Fredriksen-Goldsen and Muraco 2010; Institute of Medicine 2011). Although the reliability of these estimates is limited by problems with scientific methodology (an issue given some attention in the section "Demographics" later in this chapter), there is general agreement that the same rapidly increasing proportion of older individuals being observed in the general population is also occurring in the LGBT population. With this understanding, there is no question that providing culturally competent mental health care for older LGBT individuals will take on even greater importance in the future.

When thinking about the mental health care of older members of the LGBT community, it is important to remember the diversity that exists within this community. The members of the LGBT community are connected by their membership in one or more sexual minority communities and the potential for shared negative experiences that sexual and gender minority status confers. On the other hand, the most pertinent health issues for someone who has never come out of the closet may not be the same as they would be for individuals who have lived the majority of adult life with full disclosure of their sexual minority status.

In addition, members of the LGBT community are at risk for challenging life experiences due to membership in more than one minority group. Intersectional theory (Crenshaw 1991) is a relatively new attempt to understand more fully and accurately the inherent complexity of personal identity and to encourage the development of diversity-informed case conceptualizations that view the individual patient as more than the sum of his or her parts or any one personal identity marker (e.g., age, gender, race, sexual orientation).

The current age of an individual highlights some of the diversity that exists within the LGBT community. For example, LGBT Americans face clearly documented health disparities. Some of these disparities were present when these individuals were younger, others are unique to older age, and some exist because of membership in a sexual minority. In spite of recent gains in legal recognition of LGBT human rights and significant gains in societal acceptance of members of the LGBT community, it remains true that older LGBT adults grew up and developed in a much less supportive environment than did younger subpopulations of the LGBT community (Institute of Medicine 2011).

The 1950s were an era when homosexuality was officially equated with illness and depravity, and LGBT persons often were subject to negative societal judgments. During this decade, McCarthy-era witch hunts and blacklisting of suspected homosexuals occurred. The 1960s brought the Civil Rights movement, the Stonewall Riots, and the start of the Gay Liberation movement. The 1970s saw the removal of homosexuality from DSM in 1973 (American Psychiatric Association 1973) and the first National March on Washington for Lesbian and Gay Rights in 1979. For members of the LGBT community, the 1980s were defined by the catastrophic effects of the AIDS epidemic on the LGBT population, leading to the uncomfortable 1990s era of "Don't Ask, Don't Tell." It was not until 2015, with the landmark *Obergefell v. Hodges* Supreme Court decision, that same-sex couples had the legal protection of marriage across all 50 states.

Emerging research demonstrates that living through these historical events and associated shifts in the acceptance of members of sexual minority communities has understandably shaped the lives of older LGBT individuals and has led to significant generational differences between younger and older LGBT persons. The goal of this chapter is to present information relevant to providing older LGBT individuals with the best mental health care possible while keeping in mind intersectional theory and the diversity that exists within the sexual minority community.

DEFINITIONS, DEMOGRAPHICS, AND UNIQUE FEATURES

Definitions

In order to provide competent care to older members of the LGBT community, it is critical to understand the basics of sex and gender. Sex and gender have very different meanings, with *sex* indicating one's biological assignment at birth, which traditionally has been limited to a simple binary construct of male or female. The genetic distinction is made with females traditionally having two X chromosomes and males having an X chromosome and a Y chromosome. Flying in the face of the binary construct of sex, however, are individuals who are born with atypically developed sexual characteristics, referred to as *intersex*, as well as individuals with varying chromosomal differences such as Klinefelter syndrome (possessing two X chromosomes and one Y chromosome, XXY) and Turner syndrome (possessing only one X chromosome, referred to as XO) and also individuals whose sexual development differs from their chromosomal makeup, as with androgen insensitivity syndrome (in which an individual is born with X and Y chromosomes but develops female sexual characteristics).

Gender, on the other hand, is not a biological reality but is, instead, a social construct, defined by the roles, behaviors, and characteristics that society ascribes to a particular gender identity. In most societies, gender and *gender roles* have also traditionally existed in a binary form of boys and men versus girls and women. These social constructs greatly influence our thoughts, feelings, and behavior, on the basis of both the gender that is ascribed to us and our personal gender identity. Historically, in many, if not most, cultures, gender traditionally has been conceived as binary, but the modern and preferred understanding is that gender actually occurs on a spectrum. *Gender identity* refers to the sense of an individual as male, female, or something else along the gender spectrum. *Cisgender* is a term used to signify that an individual's biological sex and gender identity are the same. *Transgender* is a term used when biological sex assignment and gender identity differ. *Genderqueer* (keeping in mind that the term "queer," in general, although accepted by some, remains offensive to others, especially among older LGBT adults) or other terms such as *gender nonconforming* or *gender fluid* may be used to refer to individuals whose gender identity exists outside the traditional gender binary (American Psychological Association 2008, 2011).

Sexual orientation refers to the romantic, sexual, and/or emotional attraction an individual experiences toward men, women, both, neither, or some combination thereof. Various sexual identities and terms to describe these attractions exist, and it is widely documented that, like gender, sexual orientation exists on a spectrum. In general, *heterosexual* is used to refer to individuals who are attracted to the opposite sex, and *homosexual* is used to refer to individuals who experience attraction to the same sex. *Bisexual* is a term used to refer to individuals who have attraction to both sexes. There are a significant number of other identified sexual identities that exist outside the binary, including *pansexual* (attraction unlimited by sex, gender, or gender identity), *asexual* (a person who has no sexual feelings or desires but may experience romantic or emotional attraction), and *sexually fluid* (not identifying on any one part of the sexuality spectrum).

An individual's identified sexual orientation may differ from sexual behavior. For example, some men who identify as heterosexual also have sex with men, which has brought about the widespread medical use of the term *men who have sex with men*, shortened to MSM, in order to improve the reliability of scientific data in the arena of HIV transmission research. As a result, it is important to make this distinction and to ask patients about both self-identification and behaviors. The process by which an individual identifies a sexual orientation other than heterosexual or a gender identity that differs from the sex assigned at birth and to varying degrees expresses this sexual orientation and/or gender identity within the various layers of the community is referred to as *coming out*, short for *coming out of the closet*. This process is highly personal and varies by individual (American Psychological Association 2008, 2011).

Demographics

Reliable demographic data for LGBT individuals, including basic information about the population sizes of the various sexual minorities, has historically been understudied and therefore is limited. With the exception of a few recent and well-done research efforts, there continues to be a relative paucity of scientific literature related to gender and sexual minorities. One of the current research challenges in this area is that collected data are skewed because they capture only those individuals who are "out" or self-identify as members of the LGBT population. Another methodological issue specifically in geriatric LGBT persons includes "returning to the closet" in order to receive care and services in their advanced age (Grossman 2006), retreating "back to the invisibility that was necessary for most of their lives" (Gross 2007). With the inclusion of sexual orientation and gender identity in current and future research efforts, it is hoped that a more detailed and accurate representation of the LGBT population and subpopulations, including the geriatric subgroup, will be forthcoming.

As stated earlier, there are between 2.7 and 4 million LBGT individuals older than age 50 in the United States, with 1.1 million LGBT individuals older than 65 years (Fredriksen-Goldsen and Muraco 2010). Data from Gates and Newport (2012) indicated that the current population of LGBT adults older than age 65 in the United States is approximately 1 million. A nationwide Gallup poll in 2012 asking about sexual orientation and gender identity revealed that 2% of the geriatric respondents indicated that they were members of the LGBT community, and 6.5% refused to answer the question (Gates and Newport 2012). It is estimated that there are 48 million adults older than age 65 in the United States (Ortman et al. 2014), supporting the claim that there are approximately 1 million LGBT older adults in the country. The 6.5% nonresponse rate of the 2012 Gallup poll suggests a potential bias or accuracy problem with self-report and self-identification. Given the possibility that some older members of the LGBT community who participated in this survey may have avoided questions about sexual orientation for fear of persecution or "outing" themselves or because of concerns regarding confidentiality and safety, the actual number of older LGBT individuals in the United States could be much higher (Gates 2013; Gates and Newport 2012).

Before 2000, data regarding LGBT adults outside the U.S. Census were limited to isolated studies (Institute of Medicine 2011). Same-sex households were first captured on the U.S. Census in 1990; married versus nonmarried households were added in 2010 after many areas of the country implemented same-sex marriage (Fredriksen-Goldsen and Muraco 2010). The California Health Interview Survey in 2001 was the first large-scale survey that sought to include sexual orientation as a determinant of health outcomes (Wallace et al. 2011); the survey did not include gender identity as a determinant of health until 2015. In 2005, a component of the U.S. Census, the American Community Survey, also began collecting data on same-sex households, and these data were used with the 2006 and 2012 UCLA School of Law analyses of census data (Gates 2006, 2012). A majority of the data collected in the past decade has focused on overall population size estimation without exploring specific subgroups within the LGBT population, such as those who are older. Consequently, there are limited data about subgroups within the older LGBT population. More research is needed in order to better understand older LGBT people of color and those who identify as transgender, as well as the specific health needs of these subpopulations (Van Wagenen et al. 2013).

Values, Beliefs, and Unique Features

Historically, the values, beliefs, and unique features of members of the older LGBT community are rooted in feelings of being misunderstood, discrimination, and vulnerability to health disparities as well as advocacy, courage, and resilience. As noted earlier in this chapter, an understanding of generational differences among LGBT adults and an understanding of intersectional theory (Crenshaw 1991) are both essential to providing sensitive and optimally helpful mental health services. Older LGBT adults lived through eras when it was stigmatized, dangerous, and illegal to live "out" lives as LGBT people (Fredriksen-Goldsen and Muraco 2010; Institute of Medicine 2011). Some older LGBT adults have never been out to family members or friends or in their broader communities; some may have experienced coming out at a later age in the current era of greater acceptance; and some may have lived "out" lives but find themselves needing to go back into the closet as they face decreasing independence, a need for institutional care, and/or the end of life.

The Caring and Aging with Pride (CAP) study, a nationwide study of 2,560 LGBT adults ages 50–95, demonstrated a correlation between age and health risks and resources (Fredriksen-Goldsen et al. 2011). Participants ages 50–64 were relatively more likely to have disclosed sexual and gender identities and to have higher levels of social support but also were more likely to have had greater experience of discrimination. The oldest participants, older than age 80, had the highest rates of experiencing stigma, with the lowest rates of disclosure, social support, and discrimination. Although all LGBT people are at risk of having experienced *minority stress* in the form of stigma, victimization, and discrimination, research has revealed that the older the LGBT individual, the more likely this is to be true. Research has also indicated that minority stress is clearly linked to adverse health outcomes (Fredriksen-Goldsen et al. 2011).

Historically, older LGBT adults have faced barriers to accessing mental health care, including stigma, lower average socioeconomic status, and disparate access to insurance coverage. Older LGBT people are more likely to experience depression, with transgender older adults at particular risk. (The available scientific information about rates of mental disorders in older members of the LGBT community is summarized in the section "Literature Review of Psychiatric Disorders" later in this chapter.) Older LGBT adults seem more likely to rate their health poorly compared with their heterosexual cisgender counterparts, and they experience special health risks, including certain cancers and infectious diseases, as well as obesity and cardiovascular risk factors, depending on which gender and/or sexual minorities a patient identifies with (Fredriksen-Goldsen and Muraco 2010; Fredriksen-Goldsen et al. 2011; Institute of Medicine 2011).

The scientific literature indicates that transgender individuals, in particular, experience significant health disparities. In the largest survey of transgender individuals to date in the United States, 1 in 5 reported an incident in which a health care provider attempted to persuade or stop them from being transgender (James et al. 2016). These negative occurrences, specific to gender identity and discrimination, increase psychological distress and the likelihood of suicidality, homelessness, and sex work compared with individuals without these health care experiences (James et al. 2016). The 2015 U.S. Transgender Survey, capturing 27,715 respondents who identified as transgender, noted that 39% of transgender individuals experience significant psychological distress, 40% have attempted suicide at some point in their life, and one-third have had a negative interaction with their health care provider (James et al. 2016). These data also highlighted a significant level of discrimination and violence toward the transgender population, with 47% reporting being sexually assaulted. In addition, 30% reported homelessness at some point in their lives, and 29% were living in poverty, with an unemployment rate triple that of the general population. Despite these negative findings, 60% of respondents reported family members being supportive of their gender identity, and 68% indicated coworker support (James et al. 2016).

Although the literature describes various health disparities among older LGBT individuals, it also identifies areas of resilience, and, in spite of the challenges faced by LGBT elders across their life spans, studies overwhelmingly show that a majority of older LGBT adults are satisfied with their lives and are aging successfully (Fredriksen-Goldsen et al. 2011; Van Wagenen et al. 2013). Studies have identified strong social networks for some individuals and more volunteering and involvement with the LGBT community as characteristics that appear to positively influence health. Another concept identified by recent research is that having a "chosen family," or people considered family even though they are not biologically related, may be much more common among members of the sexual minorities than in the general population and also appears to influence health positively and to increase support (Rock et al. 2010). Living openly also can positively influence self-esteem and overall life satisfaction in older LGBT adults (Institute of Medicine 2011; Rock et al. 2010).

Newer studies have attempted to increase the scientific information available regarding older members of the LGBT community, especially in relation to the sexual behaviors and the quality of life of geriatric LGBT individuals. The National Social Life, Health, and Aging Project; the National Health Interview Survey; the National Survey of Sexual Health and Behavior; and the CAP study all have offered insightful information regarding older LGBT individuals. This information includes specific behaviors; quality of life data; information on socialization; and data on the specific, and sometimes unique, health concerns of members of the LGBT population (Fredriksen-Goldsen et al. 2011; Herbenick et al. 2010; Lindau et al. 2007; Reece et al. 2010; Suzman 2009; Waite et al. 2009; Ward et al. 2014). CAP, in particular, has provided the most recent and largest sample of older LGBT individuals to date (Fredriksen-Goldsen et al. 2011).

Promoting health and preventing illness is a component of aging that is not specific to the LGBT population but can be influenced by LGBT status. A 2013 study showed a range of LGBT seniors "surviving and thriving" versus "ailing" with various problems; some of the experiences that respondents described were directly related to LGBT status and others to general aging (Van Wagenen et al. 2013). Specifically noted was that "LGBT older adults have a distinct experience of aging stemming from shared experiences in relation to the LGBT community, the lifelong process of coming out, the experience of sexual and gender minority stress, marginalization inside and outside LGBT community, and LGBT pride and resilience" (Van Wagenen et al. 2013, p. 2).

It is important to note, however, that health beliefs and experiences of older LGBT individuals may influence physical and mental health negatively. For example, some LGBT older adults may experience "self-acceptance, optimism, will to live, self-management, relational living, and independence" while using resources and having a sense of self-determination (Emlet et al. 2011, p. 104). Others experience social isolation, multiple sources of discrimination and stigma, and loneliness; this can be further exacerbated by rejection from family, the fear of experiencing prejudice, and lack of services specific to the population (Van Wagenen et al. 2013). Social isolation and marginalization across the life span may influence older LGBT patients' beliefs regarding health and specifically may increase negative outcomes, both physically and mentally. A person's individual resiliency also influences these beliefs and outcomes (Van Wagenen et al. 2013). As noted in the subsection "Demographics," many older patients may stop self-identifying in order to receive general or health services or to avoid discrimination (Fredriksen-Goldsen and Muraco 2010; Grossman 2006; Van Wagenen et al. 2013). The next several subsections include information about the potential benefits and risks to the mental health of older LGBT community members of staying in or coming out of the closet.

The Impact on Mental Health of Being In or Out of the Closet

The process of coming out can be an emotionally stressful time for members of the LGBT community. The currently available scientific research suggests that for older members of the LGBT community, both choosing to remain in the closet and choosing to come out of the closet were and are associated with risks and benefits.

In the CAP study, it was found that 82% of older LGBT individuals experienced at least one lifetime episode of victimization, and 64% reported at least three incidents, with the most common type of violence being verbal insults, followed by physical violence and then police brutality (Fredriksen-Goldsen et al. 2011). Some individuals therefore may conceal their sexual orientation as a protective measure, and some may posit that doing so will lower their lifetime experiences of victimization; however, this actually may make them more vulnerable to the potential negative consequences of victimization and discrimination (Fredriksen-Goldsen et al. 2015). There is also concern that staying closeted and concealing one's sexual identity may prevent LGBT individuals from obtaining opportunities to strengthen their social networks and support systems and also may impede access to care, resulting in more isolated behaviors that can be harmful to their physical health (Conron et al. 2010; Dilley et al. 2010; Hatzenbuehler 2009).

Some research suggests that a higher percentage of people knowing about a person's sexuality was associated with lower lifetime suicidal ideation and was indicative of fewer negative feelings about one's sexual orientation (D'Augelli and Grossman 2001). Research using a resiliency framework to better understand the consequences of coming out found an association of positive sense of sexual identity with better mental health quality of life but also found that disclosing a sexual minority identity was negatively associated with mental health quality of life when controlling for social support and relationship status (Fredriksen-Goldsen et al. 2014). In summary, although concealing one's sexual identity may be associated with lower rates of lifetime victimization and discrimination, it may also heighten one's vulnerability to the potential negative consequences of victimization.

Ageism and the Process of Becoming "Invisible"

Another complex factor that can contribute to mental health disparities in the older LGBT population includes the perspective of age within each community. For many older gay men and transgender women, considerable emphasis is placed on physical attractiveness. Many older gay men perceive the gay community as dominated by younger men (Bergling 2004), and some report feeling "invisible" and ignored as they age (Heaphy 2004). Much of this may be attributed to the social aspect of LGBT culture, including the fact that bars have been a historically important meeting place for the community, and this bar and club culture reinforces a preference for youth. Additionally, the societal idea of the "predatory older homosexual" was prevalent in U.S. society prior to the Stonewall era (Knauer 2008). Given that older members of the LGBT community lived through this era, they may have internalized homophobia and may also have concerns that providers may be disapproving, or even overtly hostile, which, in turn, may cause older LGBT adults to retreat, reinforcing silence and isolation and impeding access to resources (Knauer 2008).

Whereas physical attractiveness and youth are valued in the gay and transgender women communities, it appears that they are less important in lesbian communities. Older lesbians are more respected for their experience and wisdom, and many lesbian communities have intergenerational friendships between older and younger lesbians and more robust intergenerational social groups (Devries et al. 2009). Of note, transgender individuals may possess unique resilience against ageism in later life. Some research suggests that because of discrimination and victimization during their middle adult years, transgender individuals incur less psychological stress due to aging compared with lesbians and gay men (Williams and Freeman 2007).

Within the LGBT community, it has also been found that having a purpose and a sense of "mattering" has been associated with successful aging. In order to better understand how a sense of purpose within the community battles against such ideas as ageism, data from the Multicenter AIDS Cohort Study examined the relationship between internalized gay ageism and depressive symptoms (Wight et al. 2015). This study found that internalized gay ageism (different from internalized homophobia) is positively associated with depressive symptoms and that mattering can partially mediate, but not buffer, this finding. They found that high levels of ageism appear to diminish one's sense of mattering, leading to higher levels of depression, and that low levels of ageism increased one's sense of mattering and decreased depressive symptoms.

Dwindling Peer Support Systems Despite Increased Need With Advancing Age

Research has indicated that in the general population, later life can be a difficult emotional time for some people, in part because their social support shrinks or becomes more difficult to access as new physical challenges emerge. Older members of the LGBT community confront the same challenges. The CAP study found that as the size of social support and social network size increased, the odds of poor general health decreased (D'Augelli and Grossman 2001; Fredriksen-Goldsen et al. 2014). Others found that having a partner as a social resource was linked with better physical and mental health among older LGBT people (Williams and Frediksen-Goldsen 2014). It also appears that having a shared community and shared identity provides a strong foundation, creating a sense of belonging and helping individuals cope with stigma and discrimination (Lyons et al. 2015). One study found that older American gay men were less likely to experience depression and anxiety when they reported high levels of support from friends (Masini and Barrett 2008). Looking specifically at the transgender community, the 2015 U.S. Transgender Survey found that 20% of respondents older than 65 years said their romantic relationships ended because of their transgender status (James et al. 2016). It was also found that the age at which individuals transitioned had an impact on acceptance or rejection by their families. The U.S. Transgender Survey showed that 68% of those who transitioned at age 35 or older experienced rejection, compared with 56% of those who transitioned younger than age 18.

"Re-closeting" to Enter Nursing Homes and During End-of-Life Care

As individuals age and experience associated changes in social and community structure, inevitably, some members of the population will rely on residential and assisted living communities for care. Data from the New York City Department of Health and Mental Hygiene 2008 Community Health Survey showed that gay and bisexual men older than 50 years were twice as likely as heterosexual men to live alone, and lesbian and bisexual women were about one-third more likely than heterosexual women to live alone (Stein et al. 2010). Additionally, LGBT elders are less likely to have adult children to take care of them during times of illness, necessitating care in either nursing homes or assisted living facilities (Stein and Bonuck 2014).

Surveys conducted by community organizations in major metropolitan cities in the United States showed that in urban settings, the overwhelming majority of lesbian and gay seniors—up to 75%—live alone, increasing their risk of isolation (Adelman et al. 2006). However, there is also evidence suggesting that older LGBT adults living in residential care homes feel that they are more likely to suffer from the impact of stigma, minority stress, and isolation (Fokkemma and Kuyper 2009); Jackson et al. 2008). This anxiety around stigma often drives the avoidance of routine health care, resulting in conditions common to older adults, such as cardiovascular illness or loss of hearing, being diagnosed later among gay seniors. This complicates patients' care and increases the need for higher levels of care outside their homes.

In a 2005 Washington State study of gays and lesbians of all ages, 73% of respondents believed that discrimination occurred in retirement care facilities, and 34% would "go into the closet" if they entered such a program (Johnson et al. 2005). Within a small sample of four people living in residential care facilities, researchers noted that these individuals voiced fear of being neglected or abused because of their sexual orientation. Given that they were already feeling physically vulnerable and separated from their emotional supports, they felt at even higher risk for maltreatment and ostracism from health care providers, as well as from other nursing home residents (Stein et al. 2010). This problem was captured by the mainstream media in the 2010 documentary *Gen Silent*, which followed LGBT people—both single people and couples—as they struggled to come to terms with death in residential care facilities away from their partners or at home with friends but lacking the support of their family.

Death and Bereavement for a Generation Emotionally Tempered by the AIDS Epidemic

When treating LGBT patients, it is important to recognize that in addition to raising difficult conversations, the experience of death and bereavement is possibly different for LGBT people compared with the general population. Research suggests that the deep and troubling legacy of AIDS-related deaths has resulted in impacts on the way grief is expressed and understood in LGBT communities (Blevins and Werth 2006). For example, some people whose partners died from AIDS-related illnesses may face particular challenges, including survivor guilt and negative impacts on self-esteem and identity. HIV-positive gay men who are growing older may also suffer from interrupted careers, rely heavily on benefits, and have reduced social networks (Owen and Catalan 2012).

Although most of the end-of-life care research within the LGBT community has been focused on gay men's experience of death and dying from HIV/AIDS (Almack et al. 2010), as the LGBT population ages, other experiences around end-of-life care are emerging, and most of these experiences do not specifically relate to HIV/AIDS. In fact, public health research has highlighted other challenges and disparities facing the aging LGBT community: Lesbians have a higher lifetime risk of breast, cervical, and ovarian cancer than do heterosexual women, and gay men have a much higher risk of anal cancer in addition to the burden of HIV-related cancers. There is also a greater risk of HIV and breast and prostate cancer for male-to-female transgender people and of ovarian, breast, and cervical cancer for female-to-male transgender people (Quinn et al. 2015).

As these new burdens of disease emerge, there is a need and drive for conversations around end-of-life care. Among health care providers, there is a general assumption of heterosexuality and gender normativity, which ultimately places the problem of disclosure on the patient or partner (Glackin and Higgins 2008). For this reason, research suggests that LGBT individuals may choose to not disclose their sexual orientation or gender identity to avoid negative bias and internalized homophobia and from fear of poor quality of care (Knochel et al. 2011; Mayer et al. 2008; Rawlings 2012; Wilkerson et al. 2011). This is especially significant when there is concern that health care providers may assume that biological family members' views should be preeminent over those of the patient's partner (Hughes and Cartwright 2014).

LITERATURE REVIEW OF PSYCHIATRIC DISORDERS

As noted previously in the subsection "Values, Beliefs, and Unique Features," older LGBT adults are a known health disparate population with higher rates of mental and medical comorbidities compared with their heterosexual peers (Fredriksen-Goldsen et al. 2014; Wallace et al. 2011). A report by the Institute of Medicine (2011) called for communities and researchers to examine the prevalence of the health disparities and risk factors specific to the older LGBT population given the relative dearth of existing scientific data. Despite this exhortation, data on the issues affecting the mental health of older LGBT adults remain scarce (Coulter et al. 2014; Fredriksen-Goldsen et al. 2014). The following paragraphs highlight significant findings from the available scientific literature regarding risk factors for mental health morbidity in older LGBT adults.

Historical Background and Risk

A wave of research has attempted to understand what risk factors place members of the older LGBT community at higher risk for depression, anxiety, and substance abuse (e.g., Institute of Medicine 2011). Most investigations have highlighted the historical, social, and cultural landscapes in which the current aging LGBT population have lived (e.g., Institute of Medicine 2011). The majority of the members of the LGBT community who are older than 65 years faced significant struggles over the course of their lives. Some of the events that shaped the lives of these individuals include 1) the beginning of the LGBT civil rights movement, starting with the Stonewall Riots in 1969; 2) the categorizing of homosexuality as a mental illness until 1973; 3) the AIDS crisis of the 1980s and 1990s; 4) the eventual broadening of media exposure of LGBT people; 4) the wider acceptance of LGBT community members; and 5) the U.S. Supreme Court ruling the Defense of Marriage Act unconstitutional in 2013, which led to the legalization of same sex marriage in all 50 states. The mental health of the current elder LGBT population has been affected by these historical events as well perennial community-bound biases, such as ageism.

Depression and Suicidality

Only a handful of large data sets exist that contain information about aging and mental health within the LGBT population. Data from the Centers for Disease Control and Prevention (Pratt and Brody 2014) and the Federal Interagency Forum on Aging-Related Statistics (2016) indicate that the estimated prevalence of major depression in the general population older than age 12 is estimated to be about 7.6% but can increase to between 12.8% and 13.7% for those who are older than 51 years. Depression has been consistently estimated to impact nearly 20% or more of LGBT older adults across studies, as compared with 1%–5% among the general older population in the United States (Institute of Medicine 2011, pp. 257–259). Similarly, a large and carefully done systematic review of mental disorders in lesbian, gay, and bisexual individuals found that both the 12-month and lifetime risks for depressive disorders were at least 1.5 times higher in members of the LGB community than in the general population (King et al. 2008). In the Urban Men's Health Study, which was conducted in four major U.S. metropolitan cities, 12% of participants age 55 and older reported a history of suicide attempt, and 22% of men older than 60 years reported symptoms of depression during the 7 days prior to the interview (Paul et al. 2002). In a 1994 survey of lesbians, more than half of the sample had thoughts about suicide and 18% had attempted suicide, but those age 55 years or older were least likely to have thought about suicide (Addis et al. 2009).

Among transgender older adults, the sample of research studies is much smaller, but these studies highlight even more striking disparities. A 2003 online questionnaire study of 1,093 transgender participants age 65 years and younger found a high prevalence of lifetime clinical depression (44.1%), anxiety (33.2%), and somatization (27.5%) (Bockting et al. 2013). A 2004–2007 New York City sample of transgender women ages 31–59 found a lifetime depression rate of 52.4%; furthermore, 53.5% had a history of suicidal ideation, and 28% had a history of suicide attempts (Nuttbrock et al. 2014).

Substance Use Disorders

There is sparse research on the rates of comorbid substance use disorders (SUDs) and substance abuse treatment in the older LGBT population. SUDs have been shown to be more prevalent among lesbian, gay, and bisexual (LGB) adults than among heterosexual adults in the United States (McCabe et al. 2009). Because there is a higher rate of SUDs in LGBT younger adults than in the general population of comparable age, it can be inferred that LGBT older adults have a higher prevalence of SUDs compared with concordant older heterosexuals (Yarns et al. 2016). Studies examining rates of alcohol use by sexual orientation from the National Alcohol Survey in 2000 have shown that both lesbians and bisexual women had higher rates of alcohol abuse and alcohol dependence compared with their heterosexual counterparts, whereas there were fewer significant differences among gay and bisexual men compared with heterosexual men (Trocki et al. 2005). In a study examining gays and lesbian ages 15–76, researchers found that an increase in age was a predictor in decreased use of ecstasy, ketamine, alcohol, and marijuana in the previous 30 days (Chow et al. 2013). In the 2015 U.S. Transgender Survey, 18% of transgender men and women older than 65 years reported that they specifically used prescription medication for "non-medical" purposes (James et al. 2016).

When looking at rates of smoking, the National Adult Tobacco Survey found higher rates of tobacco use among LGB persons than among heterosexual counterparts, but rates of use declined with age in the LGB population (Nayak et al. 2014). In the Women's Health Initiative data, researchers found that lesbian and bisexual women had the highest rates of smoking in the past and of being current smokers compared with heterosexual women of the same age group (Hughes et al. 2008). Older gay men were found to have rates of smoking lower than those of heterosexual men (34% compared with 47.6%), and bisexual men had a rate equivalent to that of heterosexual men (46%) (Bennett et al. 2015). For transgender people, the 2015 U.S. Transgender Survey found that more than 50% of transgender men and women older than 65 years reported smoking more than one pack per day (James et al. 2016).

It is important to note that although the notion of substance abuse is often linked to illicit substances, including alcohol, marijuana, opioids, and stimulants (Substance Abuse and Mental Health Services Administration 2014), there is also abuse of prescription medications, including steroid hormones and sexual stimulants (Lee 2015). The prevalence of abuse of steroid hormones and sexual stimulants in members of the LGBT community may relate to the focus on beauty and, some say, an obsession with age. The Seropositive Urban Men's Intervention Trial, which included 1,168 HIV-positive gay and bisexual men in New York City and San Francisco, examined the relationship between testosterone, Viagra, and antidepressants (Purcell et al. 2005). This study found that the use of sildenafil and testosterone was associated with being older (>45 years), belonging to white or "other" racial groups, identifying as gay, having more education, and having an AIDS diagnosis. In addition, men who were currently taking Viagra were also more likely in the past 3 months to have taken ketamine and "poppers." These findings highlight the need for further research on "club drugs" in the older LGBT population.

Neurocognitive Disorders

With the advent of antiretroviral medications, individuals with HIV are experiencing extended life spans. Long-term use of these agents is associated with various medical comorbidities that can increase the risk for neurocognitive disorders (Cahill and Valadéz 2013). Further, HIV itself can be associated with neurocognitive impairment. Management of these disorders and meeting the needs of this subset of the gay and transgender population can be particularly challenging.

TREATMENT MODALITIES

LGBT-Friendly Practice

The most important steps that providers can take to provide competent mental health treatment for older LGBT adults is to ensure that their practice environments are welcoming and inclusive. The American Medical Association and the Gay and Lesbian Medical Association have helpful tips on creating a LGBT-friendly practice, starting with providing visual cues of safety and acceptance, such as displaying LGBT health brochures and posters and posting a nondiscrimination statement in a visible area (American Medical Association 2016; Gay and Lesbian Medical Association 2016). Another important area to consider is the intake forms that new patients fill out or that patients fill out periodically to update their health records. Asking for gender identity, sexual orientation, and sexual behavior, as well as partner status, and leaving an option for "other" and ability to write in descriptors is helpful, as is requesting preferred pronouns. Ensuring that all health staff who might interact with the LGBT older adult patient are aware of gender identity; preferred names; preferred pronouns; and, if applicable, preferred name to refer to the patient's partner, will prevent biased assumptions. Having gender-neutral bathrooms available is also part of ensuring a welcoming environment.

Family of Choice

Another important facet to consider in the treatment of LGBT older adults is family, which becomes especially important as LGBT adults age and lose some functionality and independence and may need caregiving assistance. There is a concept within LGBT culture broadly known as *family of choice*, which recognizes that LGBT people are sometimes estranged from their biological families of origin, are overall less likely to be partnered than their heterosexual counterparts, up until recently may not have had legal protections within their partnerships, and are also less likely to have children or may be estranged from their children if their coming out later in life is not accepted by them. A family of choice is made up of friends and loved ones who may or may not be biologically or legally related to the individual. According to the 2010 MetLife report *Still Out, Still Aging*, 64% of LGBT older adults reported being part of a family of choice (MetLife 2010). Whereas overall, only 10% of community (non–care facility) caregiving for older adults is performed by non-family members, in the LGBT community this percentage is believed to be much higher. Within the MetLife study, 21% of older LGBT baby boomers reported caregiving, with nearly 30% caring for non-family members (Croghan et al. 2014; MetLife 2010).

Pharmacology and HIV/AIDS

When it comes to treatment of psychiatric disorders, there are certainly special considerations that must be made for all older adult patients, especially in terms of special pharmacological considerations, but within LGBT population subsets, there are some specific things to keep in mind. Although it is important to continue to work to dispel the myth that HIV strictly affects MSM, it is also important to recognize the subset of LGBT older adults who are living with HIV, including long-term survivors. HIV status impacts pharmacological treatment in terms of potential drug-drug interactions with antiretroviral medications. The fact that HIV is a part of LGBT history also plays a role in terms of psychotherapeutic considerations. AIDS survivor syndrome is a variant of trauma- and stressor-related disorders experienced by aging LGBT adults who lived through the AIDS crisis that pervaded the 1980s and 1990s in the United States and lost friends, family, and partners to the mishandled epidemic. Many of these survivors also have lived decades with HIV themselves (Broun 1998). For clinicians interested in reviewing HIV pharmacotherapeutic considerations, the American Psychiatric Association has an excellent set of fact sheets that can be found under the "Physician Resources" section of the HIV Psychiatry webpage (www.psychiatry.org/psychiatrists/practice/professional-interests/hiv-psychiatry/resources).

Psychotherapy

When it comes to psychotherapy, there are some special considerations when working with LGBT older adults as well. Conversion therapy, which aims to "convert" LGBT individuals to heterosexuality and gender-conforming behavior, has been exposed in recent years as dangerous and harmful. Although it has become a part of the public consciousness with publicized tragic deaths of LGBT youth, conversion therapy is nothing new and has been around for more than a century in one form or another. LGBT older adults may have had very negative and damaging encounters with these sham "therapies," or with mental health providers in general, over the course of their lives. This is especially true given that it was as recently as 1973 that homosexuality was removed from DSM. There are a number of guides available to psychotherapists describing how to care for LGBT older adults (www.apa.org/pi/lgbt/resources/index.aspx). An LGBT-specific therapeutic approach, affirmative psychotherapy, positively recognizes LGBT identities and relationships while bearing witness to and addressing the negative influence of homophobia, transphobia, discrimination, and heterosexism on LGBT people's lives (Rock et al. 2010).

CONCLUSION

Like the general U.S. population of older individuals, the U.S. population of older LGBT adults is rapidly expanding. Because of this dramatic shift in population demographics, the acquisition and dissemination of the best scientific information available relevant to providing older LGBT individuals with the optimal mental health care possible has never been more important. Although there remains a significant unmet need for more well-done clinical research in this area, some helpful research is already available and served as the foundation of this chapter.

Providing mental health care to older members of the LGBT community that is both culturally sensitive and specific begins with the recognition that the older members of the LGBT community are, at the very least, members of two culturally unique groups defined by their older age and their membership in a sexual minority. Many members of the older LGBT community belong to multiple cultural subgroups. As a result, intersectional theory (Crenshaw 1991) helps deepen our understanding of these individuals. In addition, knowledge of the relevant clinical terminology, such as gender identity, gender expression, and transgender; the values, beliefs, and unique features of these individuals; and the rates of various mental health disorders among members of the LGBT community is also important for the provision of optimal mental health care.

The values, beliefs, and unique features of members of the older LGBT community are rooted in shared experiences of being misunderstood, villainized, victimized, and pathologized, as well as the personal and group characteristics of courage and resilience and a tradition of advocacy. Members of the LGBT community share in common the tasks of deciding if, when, and how to come out and, especially for older members of the LGBT community, if and when to return to the closet. Many, if not most, older members of the LGBT community were significantly impacted by AIDS, and many lost large numbers of friends and loved ones to HIV-related illnesses. Although all LGBT people are at risk of having experienced minority stress, research has revealed that the older the LGBT individual, the more probable this becomes. Unfortunately, minority stress is clearly linked to adverse health outcomes (Fredriksen-Goldsen et al. 2011).

LGBT individuals are impacted by various health disparities. Older LGBT adults have higher rates of both mental and medical comorbidities compared with their heterosexual peers (Fredriksen-Goldsen et al. 2014; Wallace et al. 2011). A number of recently published studies have found higher rates of depression, anxiety, suicide attempts, and substance use disorders in LGBT older adults (Addis et al. 2009; Institute of Medicine 2011; Paul et al. 2002). For transgender older adults, the number of published research studies is much smaller, but nonetheless, they highlight even more striking disparities (Bockting et al. 2013).

As the LGBT population ages and researchers and clinicians begin to focus on struggles that may impact this community, it is important to note that some of the issues that are facing the current generation of older LGBT individuals may be unique to this cohort. Specifically, as the public health and social landscapes change and evolve, the next generation of aging LGBT community members may not endure experiences such as bereavement for those lost to HIV/AIDS and difficulty coming out in nursing homes. Other concerns, however, may remain timeless to members of the LGBT population as they age, including ageism, internalized homophobia, and substance abuse. Therefore, it is important for researchers and clinicians to remain focused on the needs of the changing LGBT population and to include them in discussions regarding research, aging, and access to health care.

KEY POINTS

- Although methodological challenges limit the reliability of current estimates of the size of the population of older LGBT adults in the United States, there is general agreement that the size supports the urgent need for additional clinical research and that the same rapid increase in the proportion of older individuals being observed in the general population is also occurring in the LGBT population.

- In spite of the well-established tradition of viewing members of the gender and sexual minorities as one group, when thinking about the mental health care of older members of the LGBT community, it is important to remember the diversity that exists within this community and that some of this diversity is related to the age of the individual and the impact that this has had on the likelihood of experiences such as rejection by family members, discrimination, harassment, and other forms of victimization.

- In the Caring and Aging with Pride study, it was found that 82% of older LGBT individuals experienced at least one lifetime episode of victimization, and 64% reported at least three incidents, with the most common type of violence being verbal insults, followed by physical violence and then police brutality.

- In order to provide competent care to older LGBT individuals, clinicians need to understand a number of key terms, including sex, gender identity, gender expression, sexual orientation, cisgender, transgender, coming out, and transitioning.

- Although the scientific literature reveals significant health disparities among older LGBT individuals, including higher rates of mental and medical comorbidities compared with their heterosexual peers, especially for transgender individuals, it also identifies areas of resilience. In spite of the challenges faced by LGBT elders across their life spans, studies overwhelmingly show that a majority of older LGBT adults are satisfied with their lives and are aging successfully.

QUESTIONS FOR FURTHER THOUGHT

1. The range believed to best reflect the number of older LGBT individuals in the United States is

    A. 100,000–500,000
    B. 1–3 million
    C. 10–20 million
    D. 25–50 million
    E. More than 50 million

2. Which statement is true regarding sex, gender identity, and gender expression?

    A. Gender expression is always the same as one's sex.
    B. Gender identity is always the same as one's sex.
    C. Research has demonstrated that there is no reason to discard a binary understanding of gender identity.
    D. Sex is the term used to identify a newborn as either male or female.
    E. These are synonymous terms used at birth to identify a newborn as either male or female.

3. Which of the following statements best describes intersectionality?

    A. By ignoring a person's membership in an older age cohort, intersectionality improves one's understanding of a person's identity.
    B. Intersectionality is a concept that discourages the development of diversity-informed case conceptualizations.
    C. Intersectionality is the term recently developed to describe the ability of members of gender or sexual minorities to interact with individuals who do not belong to a gender or sexual minority.
    D. Intersectionality is the term used to describe the odds that a member of a gender or sexual minority will meet another member of the same minority.

E. Intersectionality requires that an individual be viewed as more than the sum of his or her parts or any one personal identity marker such as age, race, or sexual orientation.

4. Which of the following statements is true regarding the experiences and challenges of older members of the LGBT community?

A. Data from the New York City Department of Health and Mental Hygiene found that lesbian and bisexual women were only about 10% more likely than heterosexual women to live alone.

B. Data from the New York City Department of Health and Mental Hygiene showed that gay and bisexual men older than 50 were much less likely than heterosexual men to be living alone.

C. When an older LGBT adult has been living out of the closet and then moves into residential care, going back into the closet is rarely a decision that seems reasonable.

D. The older the LGBT individual, the more likely that the individual has been impacted by minority stress.

E. The older the LGBT individual, the less likely that the individual has been impacted by minority stress.

SUGGESTED READINGS AND WEBSITES

Print Resources

Fredriksen-Goldsen KI, Kim HJ, Shiu C, et al: Successful aging among LGBT older adults: physical and mental health quality of life by age group. Gerontologist 55(1):154–168, 2015 25213483

Institute of Medicine: The Health of Lesbian, Gay, Bisexual, and Transgender People: Building a Foundation for Better Understanding. Washington, DC, National Academies Press, 2011

James SE, Herman JL, Rankin S, et al: The Report of the 2015 U.S. Transgender Survey. Washington, DC, National Center for Transgender Equality, 2016

Van Wagenen A, Driskell J, Bradford J: "I'm still raring to go": successful aging among lesbian, gay, bisexual, and transgender older adults. J Aging Stud 27(1):1–14, 2013 23273552

Wallace SP, Cochran SD, Durazo EM, et al: The Health of Aging Lesbian, Gay, and Bisexual Adults in California. Los Angeles, CA, UCLA Center for Health Policy Research, 2011

Web-Based Resources

Alzheimer's Association: LGBT Caregiver Concerns: Important Considerations for LGBT Caregivers. Chicago, IL, Alzheimer's Association, 2016. Available at: www.alz.org/national/documents/brochure_lgbt_caregiver.pdf. Accessed January 3, 2018.

American Medical Association: Creating an LGBTQ-Friendly Practice. Chicago, IL, American Medical Association, 2016. Available at: www.ama-assn.org/delivering-care/creating-lgbtq-friendly-practice. Accessed January 3, 2018.

American Psychological Association: Sexual Orientation and Homosexuality. Washington, DC, American Psychological Association, 2008. Available at: www.apa.org/topics/lgbt/orientation.aspx. Accessed January 3, 2018.

American Psychological Association: Transgender People, Gender Identity and Gender Expression. Washington, DC, American Psychological Association, 2011. Available at: www.apa.org/topics/lgbt/transgender.aspx.

Fredriksen-Goldsen KI, Kim HJ, Emlet CA, et al: The Aging and Health Report: Disparities and Resilience Among Lesbian, Gay, Bisexual, and Transgender Older Adults. Seattle, WA, Institute for Multigenerational Health, 2011. Available at: www.familleslgbt.org/1463149763/Fredriksen-Goldsen%202011.pdf.

National LGBT Health Education Center learning modules, available at: www.lgbthealtheducation.org

References

Addis S, Davies M, Greene G, et al: The health, social care and housing needs of lesbian, gay, bisexual and transgender older people: a review of the literature. Health Soc Care Community 17(6):647–658, 2009 19519872

Adelman M, Gurevitch J, de Vries B, Blando J: Openhouse: Community building and research in the LGBT aging population, in Lesbian, Gay, Bisexual, and Transgender Aging: Research and Clinical Perspectives. Edited by Kimmel D, Rose T, David S. New York, Columbia University Press, 2006, pp 247–264

Almack K, Seymour J, Bellamy G: Exploring the impact of sexual orientation on experiences and concerns about end of life care and on bereavement for lesbian, gay and bisexual older people. Sociology 44(5):908–992, 2010

American Medical Association: Creating an LGBTQ-Friendly Practice. 2016. Available at: www.ama-assn.org/delivering-care/creating-lgbtq-friendly-practice. Accessed January 3, 2018.

American Psychiatric Association: Diagnostic and Statistical Manual of Mental Disorders, 2nd Edition, 6th Printing. Washington, DC, American Psychiatric Association, 1973

American Psychological Association: Sexual Orientation and Homosexuality. Washington, DC, American Psychological Association, 2008. Available at: www.apa.org/topics/lgbt/orientation.aspx. Accessed January 3, 2018.

American Psychological Association: Transgender People, Gender Identity and Gender Expression. Washington, DC, American Psychological Association, 2011. Available at: www.apa.org/topics/lgbt/transgender.aspx. Accessed January 3, 2018.

Bennett K, McElroy JA, Johnson AO, et al: A persistent disparity: smoking in rural sexual and gender minorities. LGBT Health 2(1):62–70, 2015 26000317

Bergling T: Reeling in the Years: Gay Men's Perspectives on Age and Ageism. New York: Haworth, 2004

Blevins D, Werth JLJ: End of life issues for LGBT older adults, in Lesbian, Gay, Bisexual, and Transgender Aging: Research and Clinical Perspectives. Edited by Kimmel D, Rose T, David S. New York, Columbia University Press, 2006, pp 206–226

Bockting WO, Miner MH, Swinburne Romine RE, et al: Stigma, mental health, and resilience in an online sample of the US transgender population. Am J Public Health 103(5):943–951, 2013 23488522

Broun SN: Understanding "post-AIDS survivor syndrome": a record of personal experiences. AIDS Patient Care STDS 12(6):481–488, 1998 11361996

Cahill S, Valadéz R: Growing older with HIV/AIDS: new public health challenges. Am J Public Health 103(3):e7–e15, 2013 23327276

Chow C, Vallance K, Stockwell T, et al: Sexual identity and drug use harm among high-risk, active substance users. Cult Health Sex 15(3):311–326, 2013 23311592

Conron KJ, Mimiaga MJ, Landers SJ: A population-based study of sexual orientation and gender differences in adult health. Am J Public Health 100(10):1953–1960, 2010 20516373

Coulter RWS, Kenst KS, Bowen DJ, et al: Research funded by the National Institutes of Health on the health of lesbian, gay, bisexual, and transgender populations. Am J Public Health 104(2):e105–e112, 2014 24328665

Crenshaw K: Mapping the margins: intersectionality, identity politics and violence against women of color. Stanford Law Rev 43:1241–1299, 1991

Croghan CF, Moone RP, Olson AM: Friends, family, and caregiving among midlife and older lesbian, gay, bisexual, and transgender adults. J Homosex 61(1):79–102, 2014 24313254

D'Augelli AR, Grossman AH: Disclosure of sexual orientation, victimization, and mental health among lesbian, gay, and bisexual older adults. J Interpers Violence 16(10):1008–1027, 2001

Devries K, Free C, Morison L, Saewyc E: Factors associated with sexual behavior of Canadian Aboriginal youth and their implications for health promotion. Am J Public Health 99(5):855–862, 2009 18703435

Dilley JA, Simmons KW, Boysun MJ, et al: Demonstrating the importance and feasibility of including sexual orientation in public health surveys: health disparities in the Pacific Northwest. Am J Public Health 100(3):460–467, 2010 19696397

Emlet CA, Tozay S, Raveis VH: "I'm not going to die from the AIDS": resilience in aging with HIV disease. Gerontologist 51(1):101–111, 2011 20650948

Federal Interagency Forum on Aging-Related Statistics: Older Americans 2016: Key Indicators of Well-Being. Washington, DC, US Government Printing Office, August 2016

Fokkemma L, Kuyper T: The relation between social embeddedness and loneliness among older lesbian, gay, and bisexual adults in the Netherlands. Arch Sex Behav 38(2):264–275, 2009 18034297

Fredriksen-Goldsen KI, Muraco A: Aging and sexual orientation: a 25-year review of the literature. Res Aging 32(3):372–413, 2010 24098063

Fredriksen-Goldsen KI, Kim HJ, Emlet CA, et al: The Aging and Health Report: Disparities and Resilience Among Lesbian, Gay, Bisexual, and Transgender Older Adults. Seattle, WA, Institute for Multigenerational Health, 2011

Fredriksen-Goldsen KI, Simoni JM, Kim HJ, et a: The Health Equity Promotion Model: reconceptualization of lesbian, gay, bisexual, and transgender (LGBT) health disparities. Am J Orthopsychiatry 84(6):653–663, 2014 25545433

Fredriksen-Goldsen KI, Kim HJ, Shiu C, et al: Successful aging among LGBT older adults: physical and mental health quality of life by age group. Gerontologist 55(1):154–168, 2015 25213483

Fredriksen-Goldsen KI, Kim HJ, Goldsen J, et al: Addressing Social, Economic, and Health Disparities of LGBT Older Adults & Best Practices in Data Collection. Seattle, WA, LGBT+ National Aging Research Center, University of Washington, 2016

Gates GJ: Same-Sex Couples and the Gay, Lesbian, Bisexual Population: New Estimates From the American Community Survey. Los Angeles, CA, Williams Institute at UCLA College of Law, 2006

Gates GJ: Same-Sex and Different-Sex Couples in the American Community Survey: 2005–2011. Los Angeles, CA, Williams Institute at UCLA College of Law, 2012

Gates GJ: Demographics and LGBT health. J Health Soc Behav 54(1):72–74, 2013 23475741

Gates GJ, Newport FM: Special Report: 3.4% of U.S. Adults Identify as LGBT. Washington, DC, Gallup, 2012. Available at: http://news.gallup.com/poll/158066/special-report-adults-identify-lgbt.aspx. Accessed March 9, 2018.

Gay and Lesbian Medical Association: Guidelines for Care of Lesbian, Gay, Bisexual, and Transgender Patients. Washington, DC, Gay and Lesbian Medical Association, 2016. Available at: www.glma.org/_data/n_0001/resources/live/Welcoming%20Environment.pdf. Accessed January 3, 2018.

Glackin M, Higgins A: The grief experience of same-sex couples within an Irish context: tacit acknowledgement. Int J Palliat Nurs 14(6):297–302, 2008 18928134

Gross J: Aging and gay, and facing prejudice in twilight. New York Times, October 9, 2007, p A1

Grossman AH: Physical and mental health of older lesbian, gay, and bisexual adults, in Lesbian, Gay, Bisexual, and Transgender Aging: Research and Clinical Perspectives. Edited by Kimmel D, Rose T, David S. New York, Columbia University Press, 2006, pp 53–69

Hatzenbuehler ML: How does sexual minority stigma "get under the skin"? A psychological mediation framework. Psychol Bull 135(5):707–730, 2009 19702379

Heaphy B, Yip A, Thompson D: Ageing in a non-heterosexual context. Ageing Soc 24:881–902, 2004

Herbenick D, Reece M, Schick V, et al: Sexual behavior in the United States: results from a national probability sample of men and women ages 14–94. J Sex Med 7(suppl 5):255–265, 2010 21029383

Hughes M, Cartwright C: LGBT people's knowledge of and preparedness to discuss end-of-life care planning options. Health Soc Care Community 22(5):545–552, 2014 24935483

Hughes TL, Johnson TP, Matthews AK: Sexual orientation and smoking: results from a multisite women's health study. Subst Use Misuse 43(8–9):1218–1239, 2008 18649240

Institute of Medicine: The Health of Lesbian, Gay, Bisexual, and Transgender People: Building a Foundation for Better Understanding. Washington, DC, National Academies Press, 2011

Jackson NC, Johnson MJ, Roberts R: The potential impact of discrimination fears of older gays, lesbians, bisexuals and transgender individuals living in small- to moderate-sized cities on long-term health care. J Homosex 54(3):325–339, 2008 18825868

James SE, Herman JL, Rankin S, et al: The Report of the 2015 U.S. Transgender Survey. Washington, DC, National Center for Transgender Equality, 2016

Johnson MJ, Jackson NC, Arnette JK, Koffmann SD: Gay and lesbian perceptions of discrimination in retirement care facilities. J Homosex 49(2):83–102, 2005 16048895

King M, Semlyen J, Tai SS, et al: A systematic review of mental disorder, suicide, and deliberate self-harm in lesbian, gay and bisexual people. BMC Psychiatry 8:70, 2008 18706118

Knauer NJ: LGBT elder law: toward equity in aging. Harvard Journal of Law and Gender 32:1, 2008

Knochel K, Quam J, Croghan C: Are old lesbian and gay people well served? Understanding the perceptions, preparation, and experiences of aging services providers. J Appl Gerontol 30:370–389, 2011

Lee SJ: Addiction and lesbian, gay, bisexual and transgender (LGBT) issues, in Textbook of Addiction Treatment: International Perspectives. Edited by el-Guebaly N, Carra G, Galanter M. Milan, Italy, Springer, 2015, pp 2139–2164

Lindau ST, Schumm LP, Laumann EO, et al: A study of sexuality and health among older adults in the United States. N Engl J Med 357(8):762–774, 2007 17715410

Lyons T, Shannon K, Pierre L, et al: A qualitative study of transgender individuals' experiences in residential addiction treatment settings: stigma and inclusivity. Subst Abuse Treat Prev Policy 10:17, 2015 25948286

Masini BE, Barrett HA: Social support as a predictor of psychological and physical well-being and lifestyle in lesbian, gay, and bisexual adults aged 50 and over. J Gay Lesbian Soc Serv 20(1/2):91–110, 2008

Mayer KH, Bradford JB, Makadon HJ, et al: Sexual and gender minority health: what we know and what needs to be done. Am J Public Health 98(6):989–995, 2008 18445789

McCabe SE, Hughes TL, Bostwick WB, et al: Sexual orientation, substance use behaviors and substance dependence in the United States. Addiction 104(8):1333–1345, 2009

MetLife: Still Out, Still Aging: The MetLife Study of Lesbian, Gay, Bisexual, and Transgender Baby Boomers. New York, MetLife Mature Market Institute, 2010. Available at: www.metlife.com/assets/cao/mmi/publications/studies/2010/mmi-still-out-still-aging.pdf. Accessed January 4, 2018.

Nayak P, Salazar LF, Kota KK, Pechacek TF: Prevalence of use and perceptions of risk of novel and other alternative tobacco products among sexual minority adults: results from an online national survey, 2014–2015. Prev Med 104:71–78, 2014 28579496

Nuttbrock L, Bockting W, Rosenblum A, et al: Gender abuse and major depression among transgender women: a prospective study of vulnerability and resilience. Am J Public Health 104(11):2191–2198, 2014 24328655

Ortman JM, Velkoff VA, Hogan H: An Aging Nation: The Older Population in the United States: Population Estimates and Projections (Current Population Reports, P25-1140). Suitland, MD, U.S. Census Bureau, May 2014. Available at: www.census.gov/prod/2014pubs/p25-1140.pdf. Accessed December 18, 2017.

Owen G, Catalan J: "We never expected this to happen": narratives of ageing with HIV among gay men living in London, UK. Cult Health Sex 14(1):59–72, 2012 22077645

Paul JP, Catania J, Pollack L, et al: Suicide attempts among gay and bisexual men: lifetime prevalence and antecedents. Am J Public Health 92(8):1338–1345, 2002 12144994

Pratt LA, Brody DJ: Depression in the U.S. household population, 2009–2012 (NCHS Data Brief No 172). Hyattsville, MD, National Center for Health Statistics, 2014

Purcell DW, Wolitski RJ, Hoff CC, et al: Predictors of the use of Viagra, testosterone, and antidepressants among HIV-seropositive gay and bisexual men. AIDS 19(suppl 1):S57–S66, 2005 15838195

Quinn GP, Sanchez JA, Sutton SK, et al: Cancer and lesbian, gay, bisexual, transgender/transsexual, and queer/questioning (LGBTQ) populations. CA Cancer J Clin 65(5):384–400, 2015 26186412

Rawlings D: End-of-life care considerations for gay, lesbian, bisexual, and transgender individuals. Int J Palliat Nurs 18(1):29–34, 2012 22306717

Reece M, Herbenick D, Schick V, et al: Background and considerations on the National Survey of Sexual Health and Behavior (NSSHB) from the investigators. J Sex Med 7(suppl 5):243–245, 2010 21029382

Rock M, Carlson TS, McGeorge CR: Does affirmative training matter? Assessing CFT students' beliefs about sexual orientation and their level of affirmative training. J Marital Fam Ther 36(2):171–184, 2010 20433594

Stein GL, Bonuck KA: Physician-patient relationships among the lesbian and gay community. J Gay Lesbian Med Assoc 5(3):87–93

Stein GL, Beckerman NL, Sherman PA: Lesbian and gay elders and long-term care: identifying the unique psychosocial perspectives and challenges. J Gerontol Soc Work 53:(5)421–435, 2010 20603752

Substance Abuse and Mental Health Services Administration: Results from the 2013 National Survey on Drug Use and Health: Summary of National Findings (NSDUH Series H-48, HHS Publ No [SMA] 14-4863). Rockville, MD, Substance Abuse and Mental Health Services Administration, 2014

Suzman R: The National Social Life, Health, and Aging Project: an introduction. J Gerontol B Psychol Sci Soc Sci 64(suppl 1):i5–i11, 2009 19837963

Trocki KF, Drabble L, Midanik L: Use of heavier drinking contexts among heterosexuals, homosexuals and bisexuals: results from a National Household Probability Survey. J Stud Alcohol 66(1):105–110, 2005 15830910

Van Wagenen A, Driskell J, Bradford J: "I'm still raring to go": successful aging among lesbian, gay, bisexual, and transgender older adults. J Aging Stud 27(1):1–14, 2013 23273552

Waite LJ, Laumann EO, Das A, et al: Sexuality: measures of partnerships, practices, attitudes, and problems in the National Social Life, Health, and Aging Study. J Gerontol B Psychol Sci Soc Sci 64(suppl 1):i56–i66, 2009 19497930

Wallace SP, Cochran SD, Durazo EM, et al: The Health of Aging Lesbian, Gay, and Bisexual Adults in California. Los Angeles, CA, UCLA Center for Health Policy Research, 2011

Ward BW, Dahlhamer JM, Galinsky AM, et al: Sexual orientation and health among U.S. adults: National Health Interview Survey, 2013. Natl Health Stat Report 15(77):1–10, 2014 25025690

Wight RG, LeBlanc AJ, Meyer IH, Harig FA: Internalized gay ageism, mattering, and depressive symptoms among midlife and older gay-identified men. Soc Sci Med 147:200–208, 2015 26588435

Wilkerson JM, Rybicki S, Barber CA, Smolenski DJ: Creating a culturally competent clinical environment for LGBT patients. J Gay Lesbian Soc Serv 23(3):376–394, 2011

Williams ME, Frederiksen-Goldsen KI: Same-sex partnerships and the health of older adults. J Community Psychol 42(5):558–570, 2014 25948876

Williams ME, Freeman PA: Transgender health: implications for aging and caregiving. J Gay Lesbian Soc Serv 18(3/4):93–108, 2007

Yarns BC, Abrams JM, Meeks TW, et al: The mental health of older LGBT adults. Curr Psychiatry Rep 18(6):60, 2016 27142205

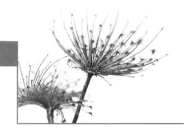

CHAPTER 9

Rural Elderly

Rebecca Radue, M.D.
Susan K. Schultz, M.D., DFAPA

Learning Objectives

Recognize the unique demographic characteristics of the rural setting that influence the provision of psychiatric services and access to care.

Identify the psychiatric disorders that have the greatest impact and symptom burden among older adults in rural areas.

Rural older adults living with mental illness, including substance use disorders, are an especially vulnerable and underserved population and one that is projected to continue to grow in the coming decades. According to the 2010 U.S. Census Bureau data, 15% of persons who live in rural locations are elderly, compared with 12% in urban areas (Bolin et al. 2015). Of this rural population, comprising 20 million people, roughly 17.2% of them—3 million people—are age 65 or older (Stewart et al. 2015). The population of rural elderly comprises both an increasing number of elderly retirees who have migrated inward as well as lifelong rural dwellers who are aging in place. The elderly rural population is further increasing as young people migrate outward toward more urban areas and away from dwindling agricultural opportunities. The elderly retirees who migrate inward are known to generally be in better physical health and have a better economic standing than the lifelong rural-dwelling elderly (Bolin et al. 2015).

There are several types of barriers to care that are faced by the rural elderly population in the United States, chief of which is lack of access to care. According to the 2010 U.S. Census Bureau data, 59 million people, or 17% of the U.S. population, live in rural or remote communities, but only 9% of physicians (of any specialty) practice in rural areas. The number of psychiatrists, not to mention geriatric psychiatrists, who are available in rural areas is at a critically low level (Council of State Governments 2011). According to survey data of more than 1,000 rural health stakeholders by the Healthy People 2020 initiative, access to care remains the number one priority for improving rural health. Mental health and mental disorders were ranked as the fourth most critical health priority, and substance abuse disorders were ranked fifth, with obesity and diabetes taking the number two and three spots, respectively (Bolin et al. 2015).

Without enough clinicians to provide specialized mental health care, including psychotherapists and prescribers, primary care providers become the default providers of mental illness care in most rural settings in the United States. Depending on their residency training program and experience, primary care physicians may have little to no specific training in mental health, geriatrics, and specifically geriatric mental health. Integrated care models are designed to help bridge some of these gaps, but rural implementation of these models is thus far limited to a few geographic areas within the country and has yet to become widespread (Kitchen et al. 2013). Even if care is present in rural areas, it may not be accessible to rural elderly given the large span of interproperty distance in rural areas compared with urban ones. Additionally, older adults may have difficulties with mobility or with accessing transportation. Last, although care may be available and accessible, it still may not be viewed as acceptable because of significant stigma associated with worries regarding maintenance of privacy and anonymity factoring into rural elders' willingness to seek and access care. Acceptability of mental health care among rural elderly will be explored further in the section "Rural Attitudes Toward Medical and Mental Illness."

To briefly describe the mental health needs among rural elders, it is estimated that 10%–25% of older adults in the rural United States meet criteria for a psychiatric diagnosis. Suicide is disproportionately high among older adults, specifically adult white males older than age 65, with significantly higher rates estimated for elderly men living in rural areas (Fiske et al. 2006; Singh and Siahpush 2002; Stewart et al. 2015).

Residents of rural areas face higher rates of suicide overall, higher rates of depression, and rates of substance abuse at least equal to those in urban areas (Carpenter-Song and Snell-Rood 2017).

DEMOGRAPHICS, VALUES, AND UNIQUE CHARACTERISTICS OF RURAL ELDERLY

It is a common misconception that rural America is predominantly white and agricultural. In fact, rural populations reflect the growing diversity of our country. Population characteristics vary by region both throughout the country and within individual states, but overall minority populations are growing within rural areas. Data from the 2010 U.S. Census showed that although racial and ethnic minorities comprise just 21% of the rural population, they contributed to 82.7% of its increase over the last 10 years (Bolin et al. 2015). It is important to note that racial and ethnic disparities in health status are even more prominent in rural areas than in urban ones (Bishop 2010; Bolin et al. 2015; Carpenter-Song and Snell Rood 2017; Erwin et al. 2010; Jones et al. 2007).

People living in rural areas are more likely to live in poverty, and this disparity has only widened as employment opportunities diminish and manufacturing is increasingly outsourced, leaving rural economies with predominantly low-wage, part-time employment opportunities (Bishop 2010; Bolin et al. 2015; Carpenter-Song and Snell-Rood 2017; Erwin et al. 2010). It is also important to note that rural residents are more likely than their urban counterparts to receive Social Security disability benefits (Erwin et al. 2010). Rural areas also feature lower levels of educational attainment, both in terms of high school graduation and postsecondary attendance and in terms of degree attainment (Erwin et al. 2010). Communities in rural settings often benefit from strong social connectedness when families stay in the same regions for generations, and there is also often a culture of self-reliance and independence. Although these values sometimes work in the favor of people living with mental illness, they can also contribute to stigma (Carpenter-Song and Snell-Rood 2017).

RURAL ATTITUDES TOWARD MEDICAL AND MENTAL ILLNESS

Among rural populations, especially agricultural communities where people have raised animals and crops and suffered the whims of weather patterns and cycles of birth and death through generations, individuals may convey a quiet resignation to the hardships of life. Underneath this is an undercurrent of endurance (Phillips and McLeroy 2004). With regard to mental illness, evidence does suggest that stigma associated with mental health services may be greater in rural versus urban populations (Hoyt et al. 1997; Stewart et al. 2015). Older studies demonstrated an inverse relationship between levels of stigma and population size, with greatest stigma in the smallest communities (Hoyt et al. 1997). Rural older adults have been shown to be more likely to see seeking mental health treatment as a sign of weakness or moral failing (Hoyt et al. 1997; Smalley et al. 2010). In a 2015 study of rural older adults and mental health stigma, researchers found that rural older adults showed higher levels of stigma and lower levels of psychological openness than older adults in urban areas, even after controlling for education, employment, and income. Interestingly, they also found that there was no difference in patients' expressed willingness to use specialty mental health care if facing significant distress (Stewart et al. 2015).

Stigma may influence rural elders' willingness to seek specialty mental health care in many ways. Older adults living in tight-knit communities may believe that mental health services are not private or confidential enough and may be worried to even have their car seen parked in the clinic lot (Hoyt et al. 1997; Smalley et al. 2010). Rural elders seem more likely to fear that they will be committed, found incompetent, and/or lose their independence if they do seek care (Smalley et al. 2010). Because of greater barriers to accessing care, compounded by stigma, rural elders are more likely to have a higher need-for-care threshold, first seeking care only when symptoms are more serious, possibly requiring more intensive treatment and leading to worse outcomes (Smalley et al. 2010).

PSYCHIATRIC CONDITIONS AMONG RURAL GERIATRIC PATIENTS

The challenges of delivering care to rural elderly have been underscored by Institute of Medicine (2005) recommendations for developing rural training tracks for primary care practice to better address known health professional shortage areas in the rural United States. As the rural population ages, health care providers will see an increase in age-related illnesses, diseases, and disabilities that will increase the demand for home, community-based, inpatient, residential, and end-of-life care. Rural residents have higher rates of chronic illness and fewer medical providers and are more likely to be uninsured. Most rural elderly receive nearly all care, including mental health care, through primary care providers because of the lack of geriatric mental health specialists in rural areas. A 2013 national workforce analysis report showed that the future demand for primary care providers to address mental health needs for rural elders will outweigh the supply projected through 2030 (U.S. Department of Health and Human Services, Health Resources and Services Administration, National Center for Health Workforce Analysis 2013).

The percentage of Medicare beneficiaries age 65 and older who live in rural areas and suffer from chronic illness exceeds the national average—more than 35% have at least one chronic condition, and almost 33% have two to three conditions (Centers for Medicare and Medicaid Services 2012). The greatest burden of mental health care is attributable to neurodegenerative disorders (i.e., dementia) such as Alzheimer's disease (Warshaw and Bragg 2014). The growing need for care related to dementia appears to be roughly the same in rural settings as elsewhere, although fewer choices of services may be available to rural communities. For example, one study prospectively evaluated dementia diagnoses in rural areas compared with urban areas in Canada; the results did not show a significant difference in prevalence of dementia in either setting (St John et al. 2016), suggesting that the risk for dementia is not increased simply by rural status. However, the lack of assess to specialized care for dementia in rural settings presents a unique disadvantage for rural elders that may hinder prompt detection as well as thwart earlier intervention and assistance in obtaining needed social services. Similar issues exist in rural areas for the detection of substance use and depression, as discussed further in the next sections.

Overall, the evidence supports that in rural settings, the hub for dementia detection and care provision through the course of illness, including behavioral care and end-stage management, is under the purview of the primary care provider. Kosteniuk et al. (2014) examined the perspectives of these care providers in a qualitative manner and demonstrated that the long-term relationships and proximity to patients and families help facilitate care that addresses the emotional and practical needs of caregivers and families. However, a need for more access to resources is a common barrier that may limit the quality of mental health care and support.

Although a large portion of dementia care is provided by family or informal caregivers, there is also a risk in the rural setting that lack of community-based home services will result in greater use of long-term care facilities for individuals with dementia, particularly those with behavioral disturbances. In rural settings, professional caregivers in long-term care facilities may report a sense of isolation and a need for education, particularly in the area of dementia management. Although most of these care providers prefer local education, rural settings often require the implementation of distance learning to provide caregiver education on the management of dementia (Morgan et al. 2011).

SUBSTANCE USE AMONG RURAL ELDERLY

In addition to the problem of dementia, national trends show that substance use is increasing among older adults, which is particularly problematic for rural areas, where treatment opportunities are sparse. One study analyzed 10 years of data in the rural state of Iowa. The study demonstrated that a growing number of older adults are entering substance abuse treatment and that this growth is likely to accelerate over time (Arndt 2010). The report "Older Iowans in Substance Use Disorder Treatment: 2010 to 2013" indicated that more than 20% of clients entering treatment were older than 50 years and differed substantially from younger adult clients (Arndt and Sahker 2014). Older clients were more likely to live alone and be widowed, thus highlighting problems of social isolation and underdetection in rural areas. It has been shown that most older adults with substance use disorders are referred from primary care for treatment, which is most relevant to the rural care setting, where primary care providers are most often the sole detection resource (Sahker et al. 2015).

Along similar lines, an interesting study conducted in rural Kentucky showed largely the same pattern of issues that increase the risk of mental health morbidity in rural elders (Zanjani et al. 2012). The researchers conducted an educational intervention and evaluation among rural elderly and also observed the particular problem of alcohol consumption. This study demonstrated that there was poor awareness of mental health diagnoses in older adults as well as a need for education in rural areas that loss of cognitive function is not a normal part of aging.

SUMMARY OF PSYCHIATRIC TREATMENT NEEDS FOR RURAL ADULTS

In general, the psychiatric conditions that have greatest negative impact for rural older adults appear to be substance use disorders as well as unmet care needs for patients with dementia and their caregivers. Further, the problem of depression in rural elderly shares similarities with the problem of dementia-related care in terms of the problems of social isolation and lack of geographic proximity to needed services. A series of guidelines has been promoted to reduce the degree of untreated depressive illness among rural older adults. These include a number of strategies geared toward better integration of mental health care within the primary care setting, where depression is most likely to be detected in older adults (Von Korff et al. 2001). For example, in the primary care setting it is possible to implement systematic procedures intended to manage the main chronic diseases of aging (e.g., hypertension). Using a similar approach, depression screening may be incorporated into this chronic care routine. Additionally, depression care managers can be embedded into the primary care setting to provide psychoeducation and promote adherence to care, which may include maintaining a registry for routine follow-up and standardized scales to measure treatment outcomes.

In addition to barriers to early detection and treatment, depression is heavily associated with social isolation in late life (Choi et al. 2015). Strategies to reduce isolation may be more challenging in rural settings. One resource in rural communities is through church involvement, pastoral services, and other sources of spiritual support. An interesting analysis in the rural Southern United States demonstrated that lack of church involvement was associated with a greater likelihood of depressive symptoms, suggesting a therapeutic effect of religious affiliation (Mitchell and Weatherly 2000).

In summary, for the rural older adult there is a pervasive problem regarding availability of mental health services. The literature to date on the types of issues that are most problematic for the rural elderly suggest that depression remains a problem that may in part be attributed to social isolation as well as primary care services that may not include depression in their repertoire of chronic disease management services. Further, the problem of dementia care presents an issue for the rural older adult, although evidence does not suggest a greater likelihood of dementia in rural communities. Rather, the need for educational outreach, particularly in complex management of dementia care in long-term facilities, presents an issue. In addition, the relative lack of community-based assistance for direct caregivers in the home is a problem in rural communities. Finally, a less well appreciated concern is the issue of undetected substance use in the older adult, most often in the form of excessive alcohol use. Substance misuse may complicate other health conditions and may require particular attention in future studies, including systematic analyses of prescription misuse. As the aging rural population continues to diversify and evolve over time, there will be many opportunities to develop innovative care strategies to meet the changing needs of this group.

KEY POINTS

- Residents of rural areas face higher rates of suicide overall, higher rates of depression, and rates of substance abuse at least equal to those of resident in urban areas.
- Rural areas feature lower levels of educational attainment and a high rate of poverty, with the areas of lowest population demonstrating the greatest stigma toward psychiatric illness.
- Psychiatric conditions that have greatest negative impact for rural older adults include substance use disorders as well as unmet care needs for patients with dementia.

QUESTIONS FOR FURTHER THOUGHT

1. True or False: Demographic features of rural America may be characterized as predominantly white and agricultural consistently over the past decade.

2. National trends regarding substance abuse suggest which of the following is true in rural populations?

    A. Substance use rates are increasing in older adults.
    B. Older adults in rural areas display lower rates of substance use than urban adults.
    C. Rural areas are demonstrating stable rates of substance use among both young and older adults.

3. Which of the following describes a problem for rural adults in seeking mental health care?

    A. Reduced availability of specialty care, particularly for dementia.
    B. High rates of stigma toward psychiatric services.
    C. Increased isolation due to geographic barriers.
    D. All of the above.

4. Which of the following providers is most likely to perform dementia evaluations in rural settings?

    A. Geriatric psychiatrist.
    B. Social worker.
    C. Primary care provider.
    D. Psychologist.
    E. Neurologist.

5. Which of the following is more likely to be true of rural residents when compared with their urban counterparts?

    A. They have higher educational attainment.
    B. They are ethnically diverse.
    C. They have full-time, high-paying jobs.
    D. They receive Social Security benefits.

SUGGESTED READINGS

Brenes GA, Danhauer SC, Lyles MF, et al: Barriers to mental health treatment in rural older adults. Am J Geriatr Psychiatry 23(11):1172–1178, 2015

Carey TS, Crotty KA, Morrissey JP, et al: Future Research Needs for the Integration of Mental Health/Substance Abuse and Primary Care: Identification of Future Research Needs from Evidence Report/Technology Assessment No 173. Rockville, MD, Agency for Healthcare Research and Quality, 2010. Available at: www.ncbi.nlm.nih.gov/books/NBK51247. Accessed January 6, 2018.

REFERENCES

Arndt S: Older Iowans Entering Substance Abuse Treatment for the First Time: 10-Year Trends (IDPH Contract#5880NA). Iowa City, IA, Iowa Consortium for Substance Abuse Research and Evaluation, 2010

Arndt S, Sahker E: Older Iowans in Substance Use Disorder Treatment: 2010 to 2013. Iowa City, IA, Iowa Consortium for Substance Abuse Research and Evaluation, 2014

Bishop B: Poverty highest in rural America, rising in recession. The Daily Yonder, December 2010. Available at: www.dailyyonder.com/poverty-highest-ruralamerica-rising-recession/2010/12/21/3098. Accessed January 7, 2018.

Bolin JN, Bellamy GR, Ferdinand AO, et al: Rural healthy people 2020: new decade, same challenges. J Rural Health 31(3):326–333, 2015 25953431

Carpenter-Song E, Snell-Rood C: The changing context of rural America: a call to examine the impact of social change on mental health and mental health care. Psychiatr Serv 68(5):503–506, 2017 27842467

Centers for Medicare and Medicaid Services: Chronic conditions: maps and charts. Baltimore, MD, Centers for Medicare and Medicaid Services 2012. Available at: www.cms.gov/Research-Statistics-Data-and-Systems/Statistics-Trends-and-Reports/Chronic-Conditions/Maps_Charts.html. Accessed January 5, 2018.

Choi H, Irwin MR, Cho HJ: Impact of social isolation on behavioral health in elderly: systematic review. World J Psychiatry 5(4):432–438, 2015 26740935

Council of State Governments: Health Care Workforce Shortages Critical in Rural America, Capitol Facts and Figures. Lexington, KY, Council of State Governments, 2011

Erwin PC, Fitzhugh EC, Brown KC, et al: Health disparities in rural areas: the interaction of race, socioeconomic status, and geography. J Health Care Poor Underserved 21(3):931–945, 2010 20693736

Fiske A, Gatz M, Hannell E: Rural suicide rates and availability of health care providers. J Community Psychol 39(5):537–543, 2006

Hoyt DR, Conger RD, Valde JG, et al: Psychological distress and help seeking in rural America. Am J Community Psychol 25(4):449–470, 1997 9338954

Institute of Medicine: Quality Though Collaboration: The Future of Rural Health. Washington, DC, National Academies Press, 2005

Jones CA, Kandel W, Parker T: Population Dynamics Are Changing the Profile of Rural America. Washington, DC, Economic Research Service, U.S. Department of Agriculture, April 2007. Available at: www.ers.usda.gov/amber-waves/2007/april/population-dynamics-are-changing-the-profile-of-rural-areas. Accessed January 5, 2018.

Kitchen KA, McKibbin CL, Wykes TL, et al: Depression treatment among rural older adults: preferences and factors influencing future service use. Clin Gerontol 36(3), 2013 24409008

Kosteniuk J, Morgan D, Innes A, et al: Who steers the ship? Rural family physicians' views on collaborative care models for patients with dementia. Prim Health Care Res Dev 15(1):104–110, 2014 23552172

Mitchell J, Weatherly D: Beyond church attendance: religiosity and mental health among rural older adults. J Cross Cult Gerontol 15(1):37–54, 2000 14618009

Morgan D, Innes A, Kosteniuk J: Dementia care in rural and remote settings: a systematic review of formal or paid care. Maturitas 68(1):17–33, 2011 21041045

Phillips CD, McLeroy KR: Health in rural America: remembering the importance of place (editorial). Am J Public Health 94(10):1661–1663, 2004 15451725

Sahker E, Schultz SK, Arndt S: Treatment of substance use disorders in older adults: implications for care delivery. J Am Geriatr Soc 63(11):2317–2323, 2015 26502741

Singh GK, Siahpush M: Increasing rural-urban gradients in US suicide mortality, 1970–1997. Am J Public Health 92(7):1161–1167, 2002 12084702

Smalley KB, Yancey CT, Warren JC, et al: Rural mental health and psychological treatment: a review for practitioners. J Clin Psychol 66(5):479–489, 2010 20222125

St John PD, Seary J, Menec VH, et al: Rural residence and risk of dementia. Can J Rural Med 21(3):73–79, 2016 27386914

Stewart H, Jameson JP, Curtin L: The relationship between stigma and self-reported willingness to use mental health services among rural and urban older adults. Psychol Serv 12(2):141–148, 2015 25602504

U.S. Department of Health and Human Services, Health Resources and Services Administration, National Center for Health Workforce Analysis: Projecting the Supply and Demand for Primary Care Practitioners Through 2020. Rockville, MD, U.S. Department of Health and Human Services, 2013

Von Korff M, Katon W, Unützer J, et al: Improving depression care: barriers, solutions, and research needs. J Fam Pract 50(6):E1, 2001 11401751

Warshaw GA, Bragg EJ: Preparing the health care workforce to care for adults with Alzheimer's disease and related dementias. Health Aff (Millwood) 33(4):633–641, 2014 24711325

Zanjani F, Davis T, Kruger T, et al: Mental health and aging initiative: intervention component effects. Rural Remote Health 12:2154, 2012 23127552

CHAPTER 10

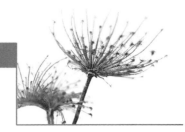

The Seventh Age

CENTENARIANS

Raya Elfadel Kheirbek, MD., M.P.H.
Yasmin Banaei, M.D.

> *All the world's a stage,*
> *And all the men and women merely players;*
> *They have their exits and their entrances;*
> *And one man in his time plays many parts,*
> *His acts being seven ages.*
>
> —*William Shakespeare,* As You Like It, *act 2, scene 7*

Learning Objectives

Recognize centenarians as one of the most rapidly growing segments of the older population, although little to nothing is known about U.S. veteran centenarians who served in World War II.

Recognize the compression of morbidity as a factor contributing to longevity.

Understand well-being as a key dimension of successful aging.

Recognize psychological strengths such as optimistic outlook to have particularly strong associations with well-being.

The impressive improvement in average life expectancy during the twentieth century is considered to be one of humanity's greatest achievements. In the early nineteenth century in nonindustrial societies, the risk of death was high at every age, and only a small proportion of people reached old age. In modern societies, most people live past middle age, and deaths are highly concentrated at older ages. Research for more recent periods shows a surprising and continuing increase in life expectancy among those age 80 and older. The World Health Organization reported that the global number of centenarians is projected to increase tenfold between 2010 and 2050 (National Institute on Aging 2011). The 2010 U.S. Census Special Reports estimated that the number of centenarians in the United States will exceed 1 million before the end of this century (Meyer 2010). Significant improvements in technological advances, public health, and prevention and treatment of disease, including the introduction of antibiotics early in the twentieth century and adoption of healthy habits at a younger age, have contributed to a significant increase in health span and life span (Willcox et al. 2008).

Interest in the centenarian population has increased steadily over the past two decades. The existing knowledge about U.S. centenarians has come primarily from studies initiated during this time, including the Georgia Centenarian Study, the New England Centenarian Study (which continues to recruit and enroll centenarians and their siblings living throughout the United States and Canada), and the Longevity Genes Project at Albert Einstein College of Medicine in New York. In addition, the Veterans Health Administration, with its long-standing adoption of the electronic medical records system, provides a unique opportunity to add to our current knowledge about this special group of people.

Generally, the findings of centenarian studies support the *compression of morbidity* hypothesis by Stanford researcher Dr. James Fries, published in the *New England Journal of Medicine* in 1980 (Fries 1980), which states that as one approaches the limit of human life span, the time in which disease develops becomes compressed toward the very end of life. The World War II combat veteran centenarians have demonstrated similar compression of morbidity and extension of health span observed in other cohorts (Kheirbek et al. 2017).

Other studies suggested that there may be multiple routes to achieving exceptional longevity (Evert et al. 2003). Three trajectories emerged from the morbidity profiles of centenarians based on health history questionnaires:

- *Survivors*—subjects diagnosed with an age-associated disease before age 80
- *Delayers*—subjects diagnosed with age-associated disease at or after age 80, beyond the average life expectancy for their birth cohort
- *Escapers*—subjects who attained their 100th birthday without a diagnosis of the 10 common age-associated diseases investigated

Although variability in average life span can be explained by both environmental factors and genetics, exceptional longevity seems to be more the result of genetics rather than environment. The Ashkenazi Jewish Centenarian Study has shown that centenarians in their study do not differ from control subjects in major risk factors such as increased body mass index, drinking, or smoking (Rajpathak et al. 2011). Although lifetime exposures in centenarians are difficult to measure in a reliable way, this analysis suggests that environmental factors have little contribution to extreme longevity, so most of the trait is likely to have a genetic basis. Several new genes linked to an exceptionally long life have been discovered: *ABO*, which is involved in determining blood type; *CDKN2B*, which regulates cell division; *APOE*, which is linked with risk for Alzheimer's disease; and *SH2B3*, which was previously found to extend life in fruit flies (Barzilai et al. 2006).

Veteran centenarians are a subgroup who benefit from integrated care provided by the Veterans Affairs health system. This group demonstrates a better health profile than the general population, with the incidence of chronic illness ranging between 0.1% and 12.8% (Kheirbek et al. 2017). Furthermore, male veteran centenarians also exhibit better health profiles relative to female veteran centenarians, which is unique given the survival advantage typically seen in women. This suggests that having a comprehensive health care system with standardized preventive screens and monitors can have positive impacts on health care outcomes.

In this chapter, we review current knowledge and focus our effort on highlighting mental health issues relevant to improving learners' competency in providing compassionate, comprehensive, and well-coordinated care for this rapidly growing elite group of survivors.

VALUES SYSTEM

Centenarians are an exceptional group of survivors who exhibit a desire to lead an autonomous life (Jopp 2016). Reducing illness burden, improving quality of life, and engaging more in social activities (as opposed to being institutionalized) are measures that not only raise life satisfaction but have also been shown in smaller-scale studies to reduce mortality (Kheirbek et al. 2016; Temel et al. 2010). The value for preserved independence underscores the need for expanding noninstitutional care programs in order to promote, rather than interfere with, independence.

Unique Psychosocial Features

Studies have identified four psychosocial features of longevity and quality life in centenarians: life events, personality, cognitive function, and resource adequacy (Gondo and Poon 2007; Poon et al. 2010). Early and late life events are known to have enduring effects in human development (Blackwell et al. 2001; Fors et al. 2009; McEniry et al. 2008). Childhood disadvantages (e.g., poor nutrition, childhood illness, social conflict) play a role in the present-day functioning of older adults, including increasing risk for cardiovascular illness and cognitive decline in later life. Multiple studies have confirmed a positive correlation between the number of children of the centenarian patient and preserved activities of daily living and an inverse correlation with loneliness (Jopp 2016; Poon et al. 2010). Predictably, centenarians with a higher number of negative life events score lower on life satisfaction (and vice versa in those with positive life events), confirming that biopsychosocial life events influence functional, mental, and physical health in the oldest old.

Global research on centenarians has found that certain personality traits predict mental health resiliency in the oldest old. Almost every centenarian study has found low levels of neuroticism but high levels of extraversion, conscientiousness, and agreeableness, as measured by the NEO Big-5 Personality Inventory (Costa and McCrae 1985). On average, centenarians are responsible, easygoing, capable, relaxed, efficient, and not prone to anxiety (Martin 2002, 2007; Samuelsson et al. 1997; Silver et al. 2001). Specifically, openness to experience correlated positively with higher scores in mental well-being, but neuroticism and conscientiousness were negatively related to mental health (Poon et al. 2010). Overall, centenarians exhibit an adaptive combination of robust personality traits that makes life enjoyable, even in the face of adversity both in early and in very late life.

Cognitive function, psychosocial variables, and physical health work in conjunction and determine quality of life among the oldest old (Poon et al. 2010). It is important to note the multidimensionality of cognition, particularly in centenarians. Social, economic, and personal resources significantly contribute to self-rated mental and physical health in advanced old age beyond the contribution of factors such as gender, race, residential setting, cognitive status, and education (Antonucci et al. 2009; Poon et al. 2010). Social resources and perceived economic status positively relate to centenarian mental health (Martin 2002; Poon et al. 2010; Randall et al. 2010). Therefore, social and economic resource adequacy are pertinent variables for understanding health and longevity.

PSYCHIATRIC DISORDERS

Despite growing global interest in centenarians, research on psychiatric illness in this population remains limited. Psychiatric disorders frequently seen in this population include late-age mood disorders and neurocognitive disorders, such as dementia. Mental health functioning is quite high among centenarians, and nearly two-thirds report moderate to high levels of life satisfaction (Adkins et al. 1996; Bishop et al. 2010; Jopp 2016; Richmond et al. 2011; Sachdev et al. 2013). This may be due in part to selective survivorship, insofar as reaching age 100 is an example of successful adaptation and expert survivorship. From an evolutionary psychology perspective, happiness would be expected among centenarians because they have effectively used resources to resolve threats to their well-being and have survived beyond advanced old age (Bishop et al. 2010; Poon et al. 2010).

Selective survivorship, however, is not the only explanation for preserved mental health. Centenarians display a positive adaptation to enormous age-related decline, suggesting a protective psychological mechanism that allows them to remain optimistic despite age-related limitations (Adkins et al. 1996; Bishop et al. 2010; Jopp 2016; Richmond et al. 2011; Sachdev et al. 2013; Samuelsson et al. 1997). Such findings counter theories of *psychological mortality*, the hypothesis that there is a systemic breakdown of psychological adaptation in advanced old age (Baltes and Smith 2003). In fact, the capacity to adapt remains surprisingly high and stable during advanced age, supporting a theory of *stability despite loss*, as measured through subjective health ratings (Jopp and Rott 2006; Staudinger et al. 1999). For example, centenarians are more likely to reflect positively on their health status, especially compared with octogenarian and nonagenarians (Idler and Benyamini 1997; Liu and Zhang 2004; Poon et al. 2007).

Self-rated health correlates significantly with functioning and mortality in the extreme old (Andersen-Ranberg et al. 2001; Idler and Benyamini 1997; Liu and Zhang 2004). Factors that lower centenarians' perceived health include increased disease burden (e.g., chest discomfort, numbness, arthritis, dizziness), loss of activities of daily living (e.g., eating, dressing, walking, bathing), and lower levels of serum albumin (Poon et al. 2010). Subjective health is one of three factors associated with individual differences in depression; the other two are relative support and loss of instrumental activities of daily living (Jopp 2016).

Unique Presentations and Assessment Tools

It is important to distinguish different dimensions of depression when assessing very old populations because common screening tools (e.g., the Geriatric Depression Scale) overemphasize age-related frailty, fatigue, and mild cognitive and physical decline, all of which may increase as a result of aging and not depression (Jang et al. 2004). When the Geriatric Depression Scale summary score is examined in isolation, centenarians falsely appear more depressed than younger old cohorts (Scheetz et al. 2012). However, scrutiny of specific items and subscales suggests that much of this is due to normative age-related changes. Therefore, a more differentiated view should be undertaken concerning depressive symptoms in the oldest old. Clinicians are recommended to use instead family longevity, neurotic personalities, social relations, activities of daily living, nutritional health behaviors, and subjective health measures as alternative ways to assess depressive symptoms (Margrett et al. 2011). In addition, the Dysphoric Mood and Hopelessness subscales rather than frailty can be used to evaluate the severity of depression in centenarians because these two subscales include the most specific symptoms of depression.

Nevertheless, there remains a need for normative data on the oldest old as a way to contextualize impaired functioning that is associated with age. Although the Mini-Mental State Examination (MMSE) has been shown to be a useful screen in assessing overall level of cognitive functioning, more specific neuropsychological instruments are able to yield more domain-specific information about an individual's cognitive functioning (Miller et al. 2010). The MMSE, Controlled Oral Word Association Test (test for verbal fluency), and Wechsler Adult Intelligence Scale Similarities subtest (test for language abilities) are significant predictors for ascertaining mental health in centenarians (beyond the effects of gender, ethnicity, residential status, and education) (Poon et al. 2010). Owing to the multidimensionality of cognition in advanced old age, assessing cognition through multiple sources (e.g., self-report, proxy ratings, interviewer observations, performance-based tests) is not only the most comprehensive assessment but also is helpful in determining the differential utility of specific cognitive tasks (Margrett et al. 2011; Poon et al. 2010).

GOALS OF CARE

Generalizations across age groups can be misleading, and the prognostic heterogeneity of the extreme old, relative to the younger old, should inform prevention and intervention efforts. The role of advance care planning is important in all age groups but is particularly urgent in this population. Psychiatrists are in a unique position to evaluate decision-making capacity and facilitate the establishment of goals for end-of-life care while the patient's decision-making capacity is intact. When evaluating goals of care for the extreme old, quality of life, happiness, and well-being are important considerations at the end of life. Treatment should encourage choice, purpose, and meaning in a way that adding life to years is as important as adding years to life (Poon et al. 2010).

It is helpful to reframe treatment as supportive care that preserves function rather than as curing a disease. Subjective health has been shown to be the strongest predictor in nearly all regression models for mental health, even over objective health. Knowing the pivotal role that subjective health plays in physical and mental well-being, treatment modalities should target preserving a sense of control, comfort, and dignity of the old. In particular, centenarians find the most benefit from person-centered care that keeps the trajectory of illness in mind and offers realistic hope in a multidimensional, holistic approach. Clinicians should pay particular attention to caregiver support and the patients' relationship with their children, if any, because those relationships play a key role in organizing or providing care along with providing meaningful experiences for centenarians. With the knowledge that mental health predictors come from nearly all selected domains of functioning, an interdisciplinary approach that considers all dimensions of suffering has the best chance of encouraging individual choice, purpose, and meaning to assure best outcomes of care for this special group of survivors.

KEY POINTS

- Although centenarians make up a small share of the world's older population, their proportion is growing. The world's centenarian population is projected to grow eightfold by 2050, accounting for 3.7 million centenarians across the globe.

- There are several routes to achieving exceptional longevity Three types of centenarians are identified as survivors, delayers, and escapers.
- High scores in the specific personality traits of conscientiousness, extraversion, and openness are associated with extreme longevity.

Questions for Further Thought

1. True or False: Behavior plays a larger role than genetics in reaching the age of 80.

2. True or False: Behavior plays a larger role than genetics in reaching an age beyond 90.

3. True or False: Among centenarians, the personality configuration of low neuroticism, high competence, and high extraversion traits is overrepresented relative to chance.

Suggested Film and Websites

The Georgia Centenarian Study Documentary (Full Version): www.youtube.com/watch?v=nUEP8se3oUs
The Longevity Genes Project: www.einstein.yu.edu/centers/aging/longevity-genes-project
National Centenarian Awareness Project: www.adlercentenarians.org
New England Centenarian Study: www.bumc.bu.edu/centenarian
Okinawa Centenarian Study: www.okicent.org

References

Adkins G, Martin P, Poon LW: Personality traits and states as predictors of subjective well-being in centenarians, octogenarians, and sexagenarians. Psychol Aging 11(3):408–416, 1996 8893310
Andersen-Ranberg K, Vasegaard L, Jeune B: Dementia is not inevitable: a population-based study of Danish centenarians. J Gerontol B Psychol Sci Soc Sci 56(3):152–159, 2001 11316833

Antonucci TC, Birditt KS, Akiyama H: Convoys of social relations: an interdisciplinary approach, in Handbook of Theories of Aging, 2nd Edition. Edited by Bengston VL, Gans D, Putney NM, et al. New York, Springer, 2009, pp 247–260

Baltes PB, Smith J: New frontiers in the future of aging: from successful aging of the young old to the dilemmas of the fourth age. Gerontology 49(2):123–135, 2003 12574672

Barzilai N, Atzmon G, Derby CA, et al: A genotype of exceptional longevity is associated with preservation of cognitive function. Neurology 67(12):2170–2175, 2006 17190939

Bishop AJ, Martin P, MacDonald M, et al: Predicting happiness among centenarians. Gerontology 56(1):88–92, 2010 20110722

Blackwell DL, Hayward MD, Crimmins EM: Does childhood health affect chronic morbidity in later life? Soc Sci Med 52(8):1269–1284, 2001 11281409

Costa PT, McCrae RR: The NEO Personality Inventory Manual. Odessa, FL, Psychological Assessment Resources, 1985

Evert J, Lawler E, Bogan H, et al: Morbidity profiles of centenarians: survivors, delayers, and escapers. J Gerontol A Biol Sci Med Sci 58(3):232–237, 2003 12634289

Fors S, Lennartsson C, Lundberg O: Childhood living conditions, socioeconomic position in adulthood, and cognition in later life: exploring the associations. J Gerontol B Psychol Sci Soc Sci 64(6):750–757, 2009 19420323

Fries JF: Aging, natural death, and the compression of morbidity. N Engl J Med 303(3):130–135, 1980 7383070

Gondo Y, Poon LW: Cognitive function of centenarians and its influence on longevity, in Annual Review of Gerontology and Geriatrics: Biopsychosocial Approaches to Longevity. Edited by Poon LW, Perls T. New York, Springer, 2007, pp 129–149

Idler EL, Benyamini Y: Self-rated health and mortality: a review of twenty-seven community studies. J Health Soc Behav 38(1):21–37, 1997 9097506

Jang Y, Poon LW, Martin P: Individual differences in the effects of disease and disability on depressive symptoms: the role of age and subjective health. Int J Aging Hum Dev 59(2):125–137, 2004 15453141

Jopp D: Physical, cognitive, social, and mental health in near-centenarians/centenarians in NYC: findings from the Fordham Centenarian Study. BMC Geriatrics 16:1, 2016

Jopp D, Rott C: Adaptation in very old age: exploring the role of resources, beliefs, and attitudes for centenarians' happiness. Psychol Aging 21(2):266–280, 2006 16768574

Kheirbek RE, Fokar A, Moore HJ: A 108-year-old centenarian survivor of acute decompensated heart failure and acute kidney injury. J Am Med Dir Assoc 17(8):757–759, 2016 27324810

Kheirbek RE, Fokar A, Shara N, et al: Characteristics and incidence of chronic illness in community-dwelling predominantly male U.S. veteran centenarians. J Am Geriatr Soc 65(9):2100–2106, 2017 28422270

Liu G, Zhang Z: Sociodemographic differentials of the self-rated health of the oldest-old Chinese. Popul Res Policy Rev 23(2):117–133, 2004

Margrett JA, Mast BT, Isales MC, et al: Cognitive functioning and vitality among the oldest old: implications for well-being, in Understanding Well-Being in the Oldest Old. Edited by Poon LW, Cohen-Mansfield J. Cambridge, MA, Cambridge University Press, 2011, pp 186–211

Martin P: Individual and social resources predicting well-being and functioning in later years: conceptual models, research, and practice. Ageing Int 27(2):3–29, 2002

Martin P: Personality and coping among centenarians, in Annual Review of Gerontology and Geriatrics: Biopsychosocial Approaches to Longevity. Edited by Poon LW, Perls T. New York, Springer, 2007, pp 129–149

McEniry M, Palloni A, Dávila AL, et al: Early life exposure to poor nutrition and infectious diseases and its effects on the health of older Puerto Rican adults. J Gerontol B Psychol Sci Soc Sci 63(6):S337–S348, 2008 19092043

Meyer J: Centenarians: 2010 (Census Special Reports). Suitland, MD, U.S. Census Bureau, 2010. Available at: www.census.gov/prod/cen2010/reports/c2010sr-03.pdf. Accessed May 10, 2018.

Miller LS, Mitchell MB, Woodard JL, et al: Cognitive performance in centenarians and the oldest old: norms from the Georgia Centenarian Study. Neuropsychol Dev Cogn B Aging Neuropsychol Cogn 17(5):575–590, 2010 20521181

National Institute on Aging: Global Health and Aging. Bethesda, MD, National Institute on Aging, 2011. Available at www.nia.nih.gov/sites/default/files/2017-06/global_health_aging.pdf. Accessed January 8, 2018.

Poon LW, Jazwinski M, Green RC, et al: Methodological considerations in studying centenarians: lessons learned from the Georgia Centenarian Studies. Annu Rev Gerontol Geriatr 27(1):231–264, 2007 21852888

Poon LW, Martin P, Bishop A, et al: Understanding centenarians' psychosocial dynamics and their contributions to health and quality of life. Curr Gerontol Geriatr Res September 26, 2010 [Epub ahead of print] 20936141

Rajpathak SN, Liu Y, Ben-David O, et al: Lifestyle factors of people with exceptional longevity. J Am Geriatr Soc 59(8):1509–1512, 2011 21812767

Randall GK, Martin P, McDonald M, et al: Social resources and longevity: findings from the Georgia Centenarian Study. Gerontology 56(1):106–111, 2010 20110725

Richmond RL, Law J, Kay-Lambkin F: Physical, mental, and cognitive function in a convenience sample of centenarians in Australia. J Am Geriatr Soc 59(6):1080–1086, 2011 21539526

Sachdev PS, Levitan C, Crawford J, et al; Sydney Centenarian Study Team: The Sydney Centenarian Study: methodology and profile of centenarians and near-centenarians. Int Psychogeriatr 25(6):993–1005, 2013 23510643

Samuelsson E, Victor A, Tibblin G: A population study of urinary incontinence and nocturia among women aged 20–59 years. Prevalence, well-being and wish for treatment. Acta Obstet Gynecol Scand 76(1):74–80, 1997 9033249

Scheetz LT, Martin P, Poon LW: Do centenarians have higher levels of depression? Findings from the Georgia Centenarian Study. J Am Geriatr Soc 60(2):238–242, 2012 22283832

Silver MH, Jilinskaia E, Perls TT: Cognitive functional status of age-confirmed centenarians in a population-based study. J Gerontol B Psychol Sci Soc Sci 56(3):134–140, 2001 11316831

Staudinger UM, Freund AM, Linden M, et al: Self, personality, and life regulation: facets of psychological resilience in old age, in The Berlin Aging Study: Aging From 70 to 100. Edited by Baltes PB, Mayer KU. New York, Cambridge University Press, 1999, pp 302–328

Temel JS, Greer JA, Muzikansky A, et al: Early palliative care for patients with metastatic non-small-cell lung cancer. N Engl J Med 363(8):733–742, 2010 20818875

Willcox BJ, Willcox DC, Ferrucci I: Secrets of healthy aging and longevity from exceptional survivors around the globe: lessons from octogenarians to super-centenarians. J Gerontol A Biol Sci Med Sci 63(11):1181–1185, 2008 19038832

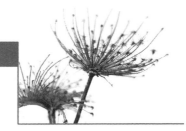

Cultural Competency and Veterans

Marilyn Horvath, M.D.

Elspeth Cameron Ritchie, M.D., M.P.H., COL (retired)

Maria D. Llorente, M.D., FAPA

Learning Objectives

Become familiar with the major wars in recent American history and how they affected different cohorts of aging veterans.

Recognize occupational and environmental exposures that veterans have endured, including extreme cold and hot weather, Agent Orange, and mefloquine.

Understand common psychological reactions to combat, including posttraumatic stress disorder, depression, and substance abuse, and the life course of these disorders as veterans age.

Understand the specific needs of older female veterans.

Why should veterans be included in a curriculum on cultural competency training for older adults? Veterans are a "minority" population who share the common experience of having served in the U.S. military and, for many, of serving overseas in conflicts and battlefields. As a result, they have unique occupational exposures that can result in long-term physical and psychological consequences that bring them to the health care system.

Most veterans do not receive their health care from the U.S. Department of Veterans Affairs (VA). In 2014, only 42% of the total veteran population of the United States was enrolled in the VA (Bagalman 2014). Many veterans seek some services in both the community health care system and the VA. Others get health care through educational (e.g., college and graduate school) clinic providers.

Additionally, in 2014, Congress passed the Veterans Access, Choice and Accountability Act ("Choice Act") in response to identified delays in access in the VA system. The Choice Act has now established a network of community providers and non-VA entities to furnish health care. The providers must maintain the same or similar credentials and licenses as VA providers and must submit to the VA a copy of any medical records related to care and services provided under the program for inclusion in the veteran's VA electronic medical record. Therefore, it is critically important that not just military and VA providers but also civilian and/or community mental health providers have a basic understanding of military and veteran culture.

MILITARY CULTURE AND COMPETENCY

When it comes to military culture and competency, if you are a civilian provider, how do you establish rapport and begin to understand what military service is like? As a start, one of the easy ways is to ask patients about their military occupational specialty (MOS) and where they have been stationed. Inquire about basic and advanced training and special skills they acquired while in the service.

Ask veteran patients when, where, and how many times they have been deployed. Do not assume that the official DD214 (discharge form) will list all their battle or deployment assignments. Learn what their military rank is or was and ask how they prefer to be addressed. Some will prefer to be addressed by rank, others prefer to be addressed by their first name. Ask what they liked best about their military service and what they were the proudest of. Do not be afraid to ask them to explain military jargon when they use it. Ask about very basic needs:

"When in combat or out on a mission, where did you get water and food? How did you shower?"

Remember that combat veterans survived war. They do not want to be viewed as victims. Treat them as battle-hardened or maybe battle-readied. Respect their service.

DEFINITIONS, TERMINOLOGY, AND HEALTH CARE SYSTEMS

Service refers to the branch of service: Army, Navy, Air Force, Coast Guard, or Marine Corps (actually part of the Department of the Navy). Correspondingly, the personnel are Soldiers, Sailors, Airmen, Coast-guardsmen, or Marines. The term *service members* refers to all of the military personnel. Active duty service members are in the military full time, and they receive care generally through the Military Health System.

Reservists include many categories of reserve service members, as well as the National Guard. Reservists usually serve 1 weekend a month and 2 weeks a year, although there are many variations. The National Guard belongs to particular states and may be mobilized in the event of state emergencies or be called up to action for war. Reservists may transition between active duty and veteran status.

As a result of the current conflicts in Iraq and Afghanistan, all reserve components have seen deployments unprecedented since World War II. Reservists' care is usually complicated because they receive health care through the Military Health System while activated but are usually not eligible for care when on inactive status. They may be eligible for care within the VA system if they have served in combat or have met other eligibility criteria. Often, they transition between the Military Health System, the VA, and civilian health care organizations.

The U.S. Census defines veterans as "men and women who have served (even for a short time), but are not currently serving, on active duty in the U.S. Army, Navy, Air Force, Marine Corps, or the Coast Guard, or who served in the U.S. Merchant Marine during World War II" (U.S. Census Bureau 2017). The term *combat veteran* is used for both active duty service members and those no longer on active duty who have served in conflict zones.

To be eligible for federal VA benefits (including health care), however, a veteran is defined as a "person who served in the active military, naval, or air service, and who was discharged or released therefrom under conditions other than dishonorable" [38 USC §101(2) 2017]. To receive health care through the VA, veterans must meet eligibility requirements, which include, but are not limited to, the type of discharge from previous military service, income, and presence of military-related disabilities.

The military health care system is separate and distinct from the VA health care system. The Military Health System is administered by and through the U.S. Department of Defense and consists mainly of the direct health care system, offered through hospitals and clinics on military posts, and the purchased care system, commonly known as TRICARE. Technically, they are all one system, but many differences do exist. For example, the providers on base may be active duty themselves, or they may be civilian employees or contractors. The providers in the purchased care system are all civilians. The base facilities see mainly active duty personnel, and retirees and dependents can be seen, but only if space is available. Retirees and dependents are often referred through the purchased care system (Ritchie 2014).

According to various regulations, service members need to be physically and mentally fit for duty (U.S. Department of the Army 2017). The medical/physical evaluation board process, now called the Integrated Disability Evaluation System (IDES), is complex. Service members may be hesitant to proceed with a medical evaluation board for various reasons, even though going through the process could offer both military and VA benefits (U.S. Department of Veterans Affairs 2011). The board process itself might be viewed as overwhelming and confusing, often at a time when the service member is also having to cope with a medical illness.

If a service member has a severe mental illness, he or she usually will receive a medical evaluation board to determine fitness for duty. If found unfit, the service member may be medically discharged or medically retired, depending on the severity of the condition. The type of discharge can significantly impact disability and health care benefits after military service. A medical discharge is separation from military service (after fewer than 8 years of military service) due to an illness that results in the individual being found to be unfit for duty, and as such, the person is not entitled to a pension. A medical retirement occurs if the person is found unfit, the disability is rated at least at 30%, and/or the service member has 20 years of military service.

A diagnosis of posttraumatic stress disorder (PTSD) does not necessarily lead to a medical discharge. If the service member responds to treatment, fitness for duty may be restored. Alternatively, he or she may be administratively discharged without benefits. Service members may or may not want a medical evaluation board, which could offer both benefits and potential shame.

DEMOGRAPHICS

Veterans come from different ethnocultural and socioeconomic backgrounds, which adds to the diversity of this population. Each individual has his or her own personal story, struggles, strengths, and values. Veterans' service, conflict, and combat experiences are equally diverse.

Presently, there are more than 20 million veterans in the United States. The majority are non-Hispanic white (78%) men (91.5%). The largest minority representations are African American (11.6%) and Hispanic (6.4%). Veterans age 65 and older are the largest age group, numbering nearly 9.5 million, and most present-day veterans served during the Vietnam era (Table 11–1).

TABLE 11–1. Veterans by period of service

Period of service	Total number
World War II	591,492
Korean War	926,432
Vietnam era	5,688,114
Pre-9/11	3,623,707
Post-9/11	4,709,095
Peacetime/other	4,626,785

Source. U.S. Department of Veterans Affairs 2015a

FEMALE SERVICE MEMBERS

Women have held military roles dating back to the Revolutionary War. Back then, their most prominent roles were as nurses, cooks, and support staff. It was not until the latter part of World War I that women were allowed to officially join the military. During World War II, more than 400,000 women served in the military. Some served at home, whereas others worked as mechanics, ambulance drivers, administrators, or nurses and in other noncombat roles. Although women did not have formal combat roles, 83 nurses (67 Army and 16 Navy) were taken captive and held as prisoners of war by Japan during World War II (Wilson 1996). Most women veterans today served during the second Gulf War or post-9/11 (U.S. Department of Veterans Affairs 2016a).

Approximately 15% of the active military are female. At present, 17% of National Guard/Reserves and 20% of new recruits are women. The recent wars in Iraq and Afghanistan have engendered a growing population of female veterans seeking health care through the VA. Thus, women are among the fastest-growing segments of new users of VA health care; more than 56% of women returning from Iraq and Afghanistan elected to use the VA (U.S. Department of Veterans Affairs 2012).

When compared with their male counterparts, today's women veterans are younger, are more racially and ethnically diverse, are less likely to be married, and have lower median incomes (particularly after age 65), despite having attained a higher education. Women veterans are more likely to work in management, professional, and sales or office industries. They are also more likely than male veterans to be employed by the government. Compared with women nonveterans, women veterans have higher median incomes; are more likely to work for the government; are less likely to be self-employed; have higher educational attainment; and are less likely to be uninsured, have no income, or be in poverty (U.S. Department of Labor 2014).

HISTORICAL PERSPECTIVES AND MILITARY SERVICE

Society's perceptions about war and the country's involvement in a given conflict is another important factor that can play a role in the psychological well-being of a veteran. Some conflicts were accepted and lauded as noble causes by society, whereas others were opposed, leading to disillusionment.

World War II veterans returned home as heroes. Parades were given in their honor, bands played, flags and banners flew in their honor, and society embraced them. Vietnam veterans reported a very different experience on returning from combat. They were called "baby killers," were spat on and ostracized when they came home, and were advised to not wear their uniforms in the United States. Today, we have a much better understanding of the importance of social support in recovery from psychiatric illnesses, particularly those associated with trauma exposures.

Combat-related experiences and exposure to specific environmental hazards can also significantly impact the health and functioning of our veteran community and their families. Some problems may be transient, whereas others progress to more chronic debilitating medical conditions that can impact veterans' quality of life and lead to financial burden. Because veterans from World War II, the Korean War, and the Vietnam War represent the older-than-65 age group, these groups receive special review in this section. Additional materials regarding issues to anticipate in the younger Gulf War and post-9/11 group are also included.

World War II: The Second World War

September 1, 1939 to September 2, 1945 (theaters of combat: Europe, Pacific, Atlantic, Southeast Asia, China, Middle East, Mediterranean, and Northern Africa)

Between the First and Second World Wars, there was significant instability worldwide. In the United States, the day the stock market crashed, October 29, 1929 ("Black Tuesday"), marked the beginning of the Great Depression. Banks closed, people and businesses declared bankruptcy, and workers lost their jobs. Mother Nature's assault on the Great Plains brought significant drought and dust storms, causing foreclosures on many farms after the farmers lost their crops. Then came the shock and horror of the bombing of Pearl Harbor, opening the door for the United States to enter World War II.

Once the United States was involved in the war, both people and industry became essential to the war effort. Weapons, artillery, ships, and airplanes were needed quickly. The vast majority of the male population either volunteered or were drafted into military service, and as a result, women entered the labor force on the home front to keep the factories productive. Food needed to be grown both for the home front and to be sent overseas. The Great Depression ended, and major changes in technology occurred, laying the groundwork for postwar social changes such as the civil rights movement, the women's rights movement, and space exploration.

In 1940, the United States implemented the Selective Training and Service Act of 1940, which required all men between the ages of 18 and 35 to register for the draft. This was the first peacetime draft in U.S. history. Individuals selected from the draft lottery were required to serve at least 1 year in the armed forces. When the United States entered World War II, the law was changed, and all men between 18 and 65 were required to register. These terms extended through the duration of the fighting. By the end of 1945, 50 million men between the ages of 18 and 45 had registered for the draft, and 10 million had been inducted into the military. Some young men forged documents or obtained parental consent and joined at a younger age. Fifteen was the youngest age reported. During this period, 16.5 million men and women served in the armed forces (CNN staff 2013).

Minorities comprised approximately 1.5 million registrants. Of these, more than a million were African Americans who contributed greatly to the manpower needs of the armed forces. Other ethnic groups who registered included Chinese, Japanese, Filipinos, American Indians, and Hispanics (predominantly Puerto Ricans and, to a lesser extent, Mexicans) (U.S. Army Center of Military History 2003).

Korean War: The Forgotten War

June 25, 1950 to July 27, 1953

In 1910, Japan annexed Korea as a formal colony. Koreans were forced to adopt Japanese culture; change their names to Japanese names; and practice the main Japanese religion, Shinto. During World War II, Japan used Korea for its agricultural capabilities and resources, and Korea became a labor camp for Japan. After World War II, the United States and the Soviet Union shared control of the Korean Peninsula, dividing the country at the 38th parallel, with the Soviets assuming control over the North and the United States controlling the South.

Tensions between the North and South grew after the United States announced it had no interest in Korea because it had no geopolitical significance. North Korea, supported by the Soviets, invaded the South. This act was viewed as aggressive by the United States and as a means for the Soviet Union to spread. As a result, in September 1950, the United States mounted a surprise amphibious landing that forced the North Koreans to flee back past the 38th parallel. This prompted a warning from Communist China that moving farther north and close to their border would be considered an act of war. U.S. troops returned to the 38th parallel. American service members became entrenched in Korea for nearly 3 years, and thousands of Americans lost their lives before an armistice was reached.

Vietnam War: The Jungle War

November 1, 1965 to April 30, 1975

After Japan surrendered to the United States, ending World War II, China's influence and communist policies began to spread in Vietnam. The country was divided into North and South at the 17th parallel, which was intended to be a temporary division until elections could be scheduled, but the elections never occurred. The North Vietnamese army, supported by China and the Soviet Union, advanced toward the South Vietnamese, who were supported by the United States, South Korea, Australia, and other anticommunist allies. Involvement by the United States was in large part related to the prevailing fear of the spread of communism. A prominent theory, the Domino Theory, speculated that if one country in a region came under the influence of communism, then the surrounding countries would soon follow (Leeson and Dean 2009).

The Vietnam War was one of the longest wars in United States history, cost billions of dollars, and sacrificed the lives of almost 60,000 Americans. This war was also the first time that Americans faced guerrilla tactics in the battlefield. Not only did troops have the regular North Vietnamese army with whom to contend, but they also had to fight the Viet Cong (VC). The VC were former South Vietnamese nationalists who resettled in the North following the end of the Indochina War between France and Vietnam.

These individuals received military training from the North and were sent back to the South along the Ho Chi Minh trail to conduct guerrilla warfare. Identifying the enemy presented a significant problem for the military because peasants living in surrounding villages would provide services (e.g., laundry, cooking) during the daytime and then function as guerrilla fighters at night, supporting VC troops. The Americans and allied forces conducted search and destroy missions in these villages, looking for signs of the enemy. Villages supporting the VC were torched to the ground, civilians were killed, and munitions were confiscated. Unconventional tactics were used by the regular North Vietnamese army and the VC and included ambush attacks, land mines and other booby traps, and an intricate system of underground tunnels.

In 1968, the Tet Offensive, a massive assault on the South by the VC, included an attempted takeover of the U.S. embassy in Saigon. The war escalated. During the early stages of the war, there was American support, but as the war dragged on and the media broadcasted daily news of young Americans returning home in body bags, American home front support wavered. This lack of public support led to antiwar movements and protests, including overt hostility toward returning troops.

Recent Conflicts

Approximately 2.7 million service members have served in the conflicts that have occurred since hijackers crashed planes into the World Trade Center and the Pentagon on September 11, 2001. Initially, the war campaign in Iraq was referred to as Operation Iraqi Freedom, and the campaign in Afghanistan was referred to as Operation Enduring Freedom. During subsequent years, both campaigns were combined under a new term, Operation New Dawn.

American service members have served in many other conflicts, including the first Gulf War (Desert Storm) and conflicts in Haiti, Somalia, and Bosnia. The latter three conflicts are often referred to as Operations Other than War. In addition, there have been many humanitarian missions that service members have deployed to, such as relief efforts for the tsunami in 2004 and recent operations dealing with Ebola in West Africa. These are not considered combat operations but are shared experiences with related and unique occupational exposures and hazards.

This newest generation of veterans is characterized by an increased number of reservists and National Guard members who served in combat zones; a higher proportion of women; and different patterns of injuries, such as multiple injuries from explosions, than were seen among veterans of previous wars. Of particular concern is the large number of veterans with traumatic brain injuries (TBIs) and possible long-term sequelae.

WAR-RELATED OCCUPATIONAL EXPOSURES

Because of the nature of job assignments, veterans may be exposed during their military service to a range of unique environmental, chemical, and occupational hazards that have been associated with acute and chronic health problems. Frostbite, nonfreezing cold injuries, trench foot, and hypothermia were frequent occurrences during the Battle of the Bulge in World War II when temperatures dropped below zero. More than 90% of Korean War veterans suffered frostbite, and 100% of those who served in the Chosin Reservoir (where temperatures could drop to 100 degrees below zero with wind chill) suffered cold injury. Health problems from cold injuries are seen acutely (including loss of fingers and toes), but long-term consequences occur as well and include arthritis, neurological symptoms (extremity pain, tingling, and numbness), vascular injury, and even skin cancer (U.S. Department of Veterans Affairs 2017).

Mustard gas, a chemical weapon used during World Wars I and II, causes severe burning of the skin, eyes, and respiratory tract depending on the amount of exposure and length of contact. Development of pus-filled blisters and stripping of the mucous membranes of the eyes, nose, and respiratory tract could lead victims to experience temporary or permanent blindness and disfigurement as a result of the chemical burns and predisposed those exposed to chronic respiratory diseases or infections, which could be fatal. Service members have volunteered to participate in studies to examine the effects on humans of exposure to low-level mustard gas. Although one longitudinal study found no increased risk of mortality (Bullman and Kang 2000), others have reported an association with certain types of cancer (Hosseini-khalili et al. 2009).

Service members historically have been exposed to epidemics of influenza, typhus, malaria, and yellow fever. This eventually led to the development and mass production of immunizations in an effort to contain and prevent disease outbreaks. The increase in immunizations had its own unanticipated consequences when thousands of people developed vaccine-related hepatitis.

Other occupational hazards include exposure to high-intensity noise and vibration, which are associated with hearing loss and tinnitus. Veterans often work in close proximity to gunfire, explosions, or rocket fire or work on jet engines or other machinery that operate at high volumes. As these veterans age, further hearing loss can contribute to health problems, including loss of balance and dizziness, and can lead to falls. Such health problems subsequently can lead to isolation and lower socialization and can mimic cognitive impairment. Importantly, hearing loss can also lead to safety concerns such as not being able to hear alarms or sirens in cases of emergencies.

Veterans who served with the U.S. occupation forces in Hiroshima and Nagasaki after the detonation of the atomic bombs and prisoners of war in close proximity to those cities are referred to as *atomic veterans,* as are veterans who were exposed to ionizing radiation during nuclear testing. Because of the exposure to ionizing radiation, these veterans are at greater risk for developing specific cancers: all forms of leukemia except chronic lymphocytic leukemia; cancer of the thyroid, bone, brain, breast, colon, lung, ovary, pharynx, esophagus, stomach, small intestine, pancreas, bile ducts, gall bladder, salivary gland, and urinary tract; lymphomas (except Hodgkin's disease); multiple myeloma; primary liver cancer; and bronchioalveolar carcinoma. Other diseases associated with radiation exposure include nonmalignant thyroid nodular disease, parathyroid adenoma, and posterior subcapsular cataracts (U.S. Department of Veterans Affairs 2015b).

During the Vietnam War, troops were exposed to various formulations of herbicides that were sprayed over acres of land around roads, rivers, and military bases from 1962 to 1975 (U.S. Department of Veterans Affairs 2015c). This defoliation program was aimed at destroying the forest and jungle cover used by the enemy for protection. More than 19 million gallons of these herbicides were sprayed over 4.5 million acres of land. Agents White, Purple, Pink, Green, and Blue "Rainbow Herbicides" were formulations used, but the most commonly used, and most effective of these, was Agent Orange, named for the orange stripe painted on the 55-gallon drums in which the mixture was stored (History Channel 2015). Agent Orange contains small traces of 2,3,7,8-tetra-chlorodibenzo-*p*-dioxin, an unwanted by-product, commonly known as dioxin, that is highly toxic in minute doses. It is now a known carcinogen, and human exposure to this chemical is associated with many health conditions, including severe birth defects. According to the Centers for Disease Control and Prevention and the U.S. Department of Health and Human Services Agency for Toxic Substances and Disease Registry (www.atsdr.cdc.gov), the most noted health effect in people exposed to large amounts of dioxin is chloracne, a severe skin disease with acne-like lesions that occur mainly on the face and upper body. Other skin effects include rashes, skin discoloration, and excessive body hair. Liver damage, alterations in glucose metabolism, and subtle changes in hormonal levels have been reported and lead to an association with diabetes mellitus. Additionally, associated diseases include early-onset peripheral neuropathy, Parkinson's disease, ischemic heart disease, multiple myeloma, Hodgkin's and non-Hodgkin's lymphomas, amyloidosis, porphyria cutanea tarda, prostate cancer, respiratory cancers, and soft tissue sarcomas (U.S. Department of Veterans Affairs 2015d).

Another condition presumed to be associated with military service is amyotrophic lateral sclerosis (ALS), also known as Lou Gehrig's disease. The Institute of Medicine concluded that there is "limited and suggestive evidence of an association between military service and later development of ALS" (Institute of Medicine 2006). Risk factors identified that are possibly relevant to military service include extreme physical activity, cigarette smoking, trauma (especially fractures), exposure to lead, exposure to agricultural chemicals (herbicides, fungicides, insecticides), and environmental toxicants.

Of great concern is the high exposure to TBI during the current conflicts in Iraq and Afghanistan. A recent study found that TBI in older veterans was associated with a 60% increased risk of developing dementia during a 9-year follow-up period (Barnes et al. 2014). In addition, the antimalarial agent mefloquine (Lariam) given to large numbers of service members as a preventive measure has now been associated with many psychiatric complaints, and these side effects may even be confused with PTSD or TBI (Ritchie et al. 2013).

TRAUMA-RELATED OCCUPATIONAL EXPOSURES

Symptoms of PTSD occur following many different types of traumatic exposure, including combat, sexual assault, terrorism, crime, and disasters. However, in this section we focus on PTSD in combat veterans. Although PTSD is now a major topic in the scientific literature and the media, especially after the many years of the wars in Afghanistan and Iraq, psychological consequences of combat exposure have been described for centuries.

Psychological symptoms were first associated with combat duty during the post–Civil War era. The term *soldier's heart* described physiological and psychological symptoms experienced by soldiers returning home from the battlefield. The psychological symptoms included nostalgia and general feelings of sadness, and the physiological symptoms were mainly cardiovascular manifestations, including rapid pulse and elevated blood pressure. The symptoms were thought to be merely signs of poor discipline or morale.

The term *shell shock* or *traumatic neurosis* was used during World War I to describe the aftereffects of combat, which were recognized to be caused by the stress of battle rather than being a character weakness. Individuals with the condition were jumpy, and loud noises produced exaggerated startle reactions. During World War II, the symptoms were called *battle fatigue*, and psychiatric casualties increased 300% compared with World War I (Figley 1978). It was not until after the Vietnam War, however, that the symptoms were first conceptualized as a psychiatric disorder.

Studies of combat veterans and active duty service members who have deployed to combat theaters consistently report prevalence rates of syndromal PTSD in the range of 11%–20% (Institute of Medicine 2014; Tanielian and Jaycox 2008). According to the National Vietnam Veterans' Readjustment Study (NVVRS), it is estimated that 30% of Vietnam veterans meet criteria for PTSD at some point in their lives (Kulka et al. 1990a, 1990b), and this higher rate may be due in part to the severe treatment they received on returning home. An additional 22% of men and 21% of women Vietnam veterans have had at least subsyndromal PTSD in their lifetime. Only a small number of Vietnam veterans have attempted to seek care from mental health providers. Data from the Matsunaga Vietnam Veterans Project (Schnurr et al. 2003) found that contrary to the initial analysis of the NVVRS data, a large majority of Vietnam veterans struggle with chronic PTSD symptoms, with four out of five reporting recent symptoms when interviewed 20–25 years after Vietnam. Veterans with high levels of war zone exposure had significantly higher rates, with 35.8% of men and 17.5% of women meeting criteria for current PTSD. Both full criteria and subsyndromal PTSD have been associated with negative outcomes, including alcohol abuse or dependence, tobacco use, marital problems and divorce, increased involvement in the justice system, parenting difficulties, and suicide (Chopra et al. 2014; Durai et al. 2011).

In addition, there are medical comorbidities associated with PTSD, including hypertension; early cardiovascular disease; asthma; chronic obstructive pulmonary disease; chronic fatigue syndrome; arthritis; fibromyalgia; migraine headaches; cancer; and other respiratory, cardiovascular, gastrointestinal, or pain disorders (Sareen et al. 2007; Schnurr et al. 2000). Individuals with PTSD also report poor social support, social isolation, and higher health care utilization.

COMBAT PTSD AND AGING

The symptoms of PTSD can persist into later years, even decades after the combat experience, because this is a chronic condition that is the result of a life-changing experience. In some cases, PTSD symptoms increase with aging. This can be due to several reasons. Many veterans with PTSD volunteer to work overtime or on weekends as a coping mechanism. Once they retire, however, they no longer have work to serve as a distraction, and with more available time, they may begin to recall and ruminate about the war experience. In later life, many veterans stop consuming alcohol because of medical problems or medications. Alcohol also may have been used as a coping strategy, and when this is removed, the veteran begins to have difficulty coping. Additionally, today's news items are graphic in nature, and because of the 24-hour news cycle, one is exposed to repetitive reports of traumatic events from the entire world. This can trigger intrusive recollections in the combat veteran. Last, life-threatening medical diagnoses (such as heart attacks or cancer) can cause the veteran to feel vulnerable, rekindling fears of death that occurred on the battlefield and triggering a resurgence of PTSD symptoms.

PTSD has been associated with an increased risk of developing dementia. A large retrospective cohort study using the national VA database found a nearly twofold increased risk of developing dementia among veterans with PTSD when compared with those who did not have PTSD (Yaffe et al. 2010). In addition, a recent case series has reported that with the onset of dementia, previously controlled symptoms of PTSD may worsen (Mittal et al. 2001).

MORAL INJURY

The concept of *moral injury* is an existential condition, related to but different from PTSD, which is a medical diagnosis. In general, most authors conceptualize it as an insult caused either by shame of killing or by the guilt induced by having fellow service members die while one has survived. Although moral injury has not been well studied by the medical community, most agree that it is a corrosive condition that contributes to relationship difficulties and suicide.

SUICIDE

Suicides among U.S. Army personnel have been increasing since 2004, surpassing comparable civilian rates in 2008. They peaked in active duty troops in the last few years but are still rising in reservists. Suicides among veterans are estimated at 22 a day (U.S. Department of Veterans Affairs 2016b). Suicides are consistently highest among young white males but have been rising in older ages and females as well.

Risk factors for suicide among active duty members are well known because data are systemically collected. These factors include relationship difficulties, financial and occupational problems, pain and physical disability, and access to weapons (Black et al. 2011; Ritchie 2012). Less is known about risk factors among veterans than for those on active duty. Anecdotally, suicides among recent veterans have the same risk factors as with active duty service members. For older veterans, they seem to be related to depression, unstable housing, and substance dependence.

The National Suicide Prevention Lifeline has demonstrated effectiveness in reducing suicidality during a telephone session, with decreases in hopelessness in the following weeks (Gould et al. 2007). Veterans should be provided with the phone number for this hotline: 1-800-273-8255 (press 1).

EVIDENCE-BASED TREATMENTS

There are two forms of evidence-based treatment from well-established guidelines for the treatment of PTSD, developed by the American Psychiatric Association, the U.S. Department of Defense, and the VA: 1) pharmacotherapy or medication and 2) psychotherapy. Pharmacotherapy includes two U.S. Food and Drug Administration–approved selective serotonin reuptake inhibitors (SSRIs): paroxetine (Paxil) and sertraline (Zoloft). However, most clinicians use a wide variety of SSRIs, with the choice depending on the side-effect profile of each agent. Many other medications are also used, including second-generation antipsychotics and other standard medications for sleep. Recently, decreased PTSD-associated nightmare severity has been consistently reported with the use of prazosin in dosages ranging from 1 mg/day to 16 mg/day (Kung et al. 2012).

Evidence-based psychotherapies include 1) cognitive processing therapy, a variant of cognitive-behavioral therapy, and 2) prolonged exposure therapy. The first therapy involves telling the combat-related trauma and reframing it. The second includes reexposure to the trauma in a gradual process. A variant of exposure therapy includes virtual therapy, a computer-aided reexposure process. Eye movement desensitizing and reprocessing is also an approved treatment, although many consider it another variant of exposure therapy. These forms of treatment have been examined primarily in younger adults. A recent case described modifications in prolonged exposure therapy that were successfully used with an older combat veteran with both PTSD and mild dementia (Duax et al. 2013).

KEY POINTS

- Civilian providers will be taking care of veterans and their family members for the foreseeable future.
- It is critical to understand the diverse and unique psychiatric and cultural issues of the veteran populations.
- As veterans age, retire, develop health-related (and, in some cases, life-threatening) illnesses, and lose family members and friends, symptoms related to war experiences that recur can be addressed to alleviate symptoms.

QUESTIONS FOR FURTHER THOUGHT

1. Most present-day veterans served during which of the following eras?

   A. World War II.
   B. Korean War.
   C. Vietnam.
   D. First Gulf War.
   E. Operation Enduring Freedom/Operation Iraqi Freedom.

2. Which of the following combat occupational exposures has been associated with an increased risk of developing dementia in a 9-year follow-up period?

    A. Mustard gas.

    B. Agent Orange.

    C. Exposure to cold.

    D. Traumatic brain injury.

    E. Extreme physical activity.

3. True or False: In later life, all veterans who stop consuming alcohol demonstrate improved quality of life and fewer psychological symptoms.

4. True or False: As combat veterans age and develop dementia, symptoms of PTSD can recur.

5. Which of the following medications has been found to decrease nightmares associated with PTSD?

    A. Propranolol.

    B. Cimetidine.

    C. Amantadine.

    D. Prazocin.

    E. Quetiapine.

6. All of the following items are risk factors for suicide among active duty service members except

    A. Relationship difficulties.

    B. Access to firearms.

    C. Pain.

    D. Occupational problems.

    E. Fear of death.

SUGGESTED READINGS, WEBSITES, AND FILMS

Readings and Websites

National Academies of Sciences, Engineering, and Medicine: Noise and Military Service: Implications for Hearing Loss and Tinnitus. Washington, DC, National Academies Press, September 22, 2005. Available at: www.nationalacademies.org/hmd/Reports/2005/Noise-and-Military-Service-Implications-for-Hearing-Loss-and-Tinnitus.aspx. Accessed January 10, 2018.

National World War II Museum: Research Starters: The Draft and World War II. New Orleans, LA, National World War II Museum, 2018. Available at: www.nationalww2museum.org/learn/education/for-students/ww2-history/take-a-closer-look/draft-registration-documents.html. Accessed January 10, 2018.

U.S. Department of Veterans Affairs: America's wars fact sheet. Washington, DC, Office of Public Affairs, May 2017. Available at: www.va.gov/opa/publications/factsheets/fs_americas_wars.pdf. Accessed January 10, 2018.

U.S. Department of Veterans Affairs: VA/DoD Clinical Practice Guidelines: Management of Posttraumatic Stress Disorder and Acute Stress Disorder. Washington, DC, U.S. Department of Veterans Affairs, 2017. Available at: www.healthquality.va.gov/index.asp. Accessed January 10, 2018.

U.S. National Library of Medicine: The Wilber A. Sawyer Papers: Controlling Diseases During World War II, 1939–1944. Bethesda, MD, U.S. National Library of Medicine, 2018. Available at: https://profiles.nlm.nih.gov/ps/retrieve/Narrative/LW/p-nid/139. Accessed January 10, 2018.

War Related Illness and Injury Study Center: Evaluating veterans with environmental exposure concerns: the basics. Washington, DC, U.S. Department of Veterans Affairs, 2015. Available at: www.warrelatedillness.va.gov/education/factsheets/evaluating-veterans-with-environmental-exposure-concerns.pdf. Accessed January 10, 2018.

Films

Huston, J: Shades of Gray (Professional Medical Film series, PMF 5047), 1948. PMF was a series of technical motion pictures produced by the U.S. Army from the mid-1940s through the late 1960s. *Shades of Gray* depicted soldiers who presented with combat-related stress symptoms of varying degrees.

Kakert P: Escape From Firebase Kate, 2015. This 1-hour documentary recounts the events of an intense 3-day siege during the Vietnam War in 1969 on Firebase Kate, just off the Ho Chi Minh trail. The film depicts the consequences of the implementation of U.S. policy of Vietnamization, which called for U.S. troops to turn over the war effort to the South Vietnamese Army. The film describes the experiences and thoughts of U.S. soldiers, as well as the pilots who flew around the firebase. Audio recordings of the actual communications between air support and ground troops are part of the film.

REFERENCES

Bagalman E: The Number of Veterans That Use VA Health Care Services: A Fact Sheet. Washington, DC, Congressional Research Service, June 3, 2014. Available at: https://fas.org/sgp/crs/misc/R43579.pdf. Accessed January 10, 2018.

Barnes DE, Kaup A, Kirby KA, et al: Traumatic brain injury and risk of dementia in older veterans. Neurology 83(4):312–319, 2014 24966406

Black S, Galloway S, Bell M, et al: Prevalence and risk factors associated with suicides of Army soldiers. Mil Psychol 23:433–451, 2011

Bullman T, Kang H: A fifty year mortality follow-up study of veterans exposed to low level chemical warfare agent, mustard gas. Ann Epidemiol 10(5):333–338, 2000 10942882

Chopra MP, Zhang H, Pless Kaiser A, et al: PTSD is a chronic, fluctuating disorder affecting the mental quality of life in older adults. Am J Geriatr Psychiatry 22(1):86–97, 2014 24314889

CNN staff: By the numbers: U.S. war veterans. Atlanta, GA, CNN, 2013. Available at: www.cnn.com/2013/06/05/us/war-veterans-by-the-numbers/index.html. Accessed may 29, 2018.

Duax JM, Waldron-Perrine B, Rauch SAM, et al: Prolonged exposure therapy for a Vietnam veteran with PTSD and early-stage dementia. Cognit Behav Pract 20(1):64–73, 2013

Durai UN, Chopra MP, Coakley E, et al: Exposure to trauma and posttraumatic stress disorder symptoms in older veterans attending primary care: comorbid conditions and self-rated health status. J Am Geriatr Soc 59(6):1087–1092, 2011 21649614

Gould MS, Kalafat J, Harrismunfakh JL, et al: An evaluation of crisis hotline outcomes part 2: suicidal callers. Suicide Life Threat Behav 37(3):338–352, 2007 17579545

Figley CR: Stress Disorders Among Vietnam Veterans: Theory, Research, and Treatment. New York, Brunner-Routledge, 1978

History Channel: Agent Orange. New York, History, 2015. Available at: www.history.com/topics/vietnam-war/agent-orange. Accessed May 29, 2018.

Hosseini-khalili A, Haines DD, Modirian E, et al: Mustard gas exposure and carcinogenesis of lung. Mutat Res 678(1):1–6, 2009 19559099

Institute of Medicine: Amyotrophic Lateral Sclerosis in Veterans: Review of the Scientific Literature. Washington, DC, National Academies Press, 2006. Available at: www.nap.edu/read/11757/chapter/1#ii. Accessed January 10, 2018.

Institute of Medicine: Treatment of Posttraumatic Stress Disorder in Military and Veteran Populations. Washington, DC, National Academies Press, 2014.

Kulka RA, Schlenger WE, Fairbank JA, et al: The National Vietnam Veterans Readjustment Study: Tables of Findings and Technical Appendices. New York, Brunner/Mazel, 1990a

Kulka RA, Schlenger WE, Fairbank JA, et al: Trauma and the Vietnam War Generation: Report of Findings From the National Vietnam Veterans Readjustment Study. New York, Brunner/Mazel, 1990b

Kung S, Espinel Z, Lapid MI: Treatment of nightmares with prazosin: a systematic review. Mayo Clin Proc 87(9):890–900, 2012 22883741

Leeson PT, Dean A: The democratic domino theory. Am J Pol Sci 53(3):533–551, 2009

Mittal D, Torres R, Abashidze A, et al: Worsening of PTSD symptoms with cognitive decline: case series. J Geriatr Psychiatry Neurol 14(1):17–20, 2001 11281311

Ritchie EC: Suicides and the United States Army: perspectives from the former psychiatry consultant to the Army Surgeon General. Cerebrum, January 25, 2012. Available at: www.dana.org/Cerebrum/2012/Suicide_and_the_United_States_Army__Perspectives_from_the_Former_Psychiatry_Consultant_to_the_Army_Surgeon_General. Accessed January 12, 2018.

Ritchie EC: Military health care system and U.S. Department of Veterans Affairs: an overview, in Care of Military Service Members, Veterans, and Their Families. Edited by Cozza S, Goldenberg M, Ursano RJ. Washington, DC, American Psychiatric Publishing, 2014, pp 53–72

Ritchie EC, Nevin R, Block J: Psychiatric side effects of mefloquine: relevance to forensic psychiatry. J Am Psychiatry Law 41(2):224–235, 2013 23771936

Sareen J, Cox BJ, Stein MB, et al: Physical and mental comorbidity, disability, and suicidal behavior associated with posttraumatic stress disorder in a large community sample. Psychosom Med 69(3):242–248, 2007 17401056

Schnurr PP, Spiro A 3rd, Paris AH: Physician-diagnosed medical disorders in relation to PTSD symptoms in older male military veterans. Health Psychol 19(1):91–97, 2000 10711592

Schnurr PP, Lunney CA, Sengupta A, et al: A descriptive analysis of PTSD chronicity in Vietnam veterans. J Trauma Stress 16(6):545–553, 2003 14690351

Tanielian T, Jaycox LH (eds): Invisible Wounds of War: Psychological and Cognitive Injuries, Their Consequences, and Services to Assist Recovery. Santa Monica, CA, Rand Corporation, 2008. Available at: www.rand.org/content/dam/rand/pubs/monographs/2008/RAND_MG720.pdf. Accessed January 13, 2018.

U.S. Army Center of Military History: Minority Groups in World War II. Washington, DC, U.S Army Center of Military History, 2003. Available at: https://history.army.mil/documents/WWII/minst.htm. Accessed May 29, 2018

U.S. Census Bureau: Glossary: who are veterans? Suitland, MD, U.S. Census Bureau, April 6, 2017. Available at: www.census.gov/topics/population/veterans/about/glossary.html#par_textimage_1. Accessed January 13, 2018.

U.S. Department of the Army: Army Regulation 40-501: Standards of Medical Fitness. Fort Belvoir, VA, Army Publishing Directorate, June 14, 2017. Available at: https://armypubs.army.mil/epubs/DR_pubs/DR_a/pdf/web/ARN3801_AR40-501_Web_FINAL.pdf. Accessed January 10, 2018.

U.S. Department of Labor: Issue Brief: Women Veterans Profile. Washington, DC, Women's Bureau, 2014. Available at: www.dol.gov/wb/media/Women_Veterans_Profile.pdf. Accessed May 11, 2018.

U.S. Department of Veterans Affairs: Integrated Disability Evaluation System (IDES) Information Support Plan. Washington, DC, VLER Enterprise Program Management Office, September 2011. Available at: www.va.gov/VLER/docs/SourceDocs/IDES_ISP_v1_20110901.pdf. Accessed January 10, 2018.

U.S. Department of Veterans Affairs: Women Veterans Health Care Fact Sheet. Washington, DC, U.S. Department of Veterans Affairs, 2012. Available at: www.womenshealth.va.gov/WOMENSHEALTH/docs/WH_facts_FINAL.pdf Accessed May 29, 2018.

U.S. Department of Veterans Affairs: Veterans by Period of Service and by Children not in the Household as of 9/30/2015. 2015a. Washington, DC, U.S. Department of Veterans Affairs, Available at: www.va.gov/vetdata/docs/Quickfacts/Veterans_by_POS_and_by_Children.pdf. Accessed January 10, 2018.

U.S. Department of Veterans Affairs: Diseases Associated With Ionizing Radiation. June 3, 2015b. Available at: www.publichealth.va.gov/exposures/radiation/diseases.asp. Washington, DC, U.S. Department of Veterans Affairs, Accessed January 10, 2018.

U.S. Department of Veterans Affairs: Facts About Herbicides. U.S. Department of Veterans Affairs, 2015c. Available at: www.publichealth.va.gov/exposures/agentorange/basics.asp. Accessed May 29, 2018.

U.S. Department of Veterans Affairs: Veterans' Diseases Associated With Agent Orange. Washington, DC, U.S. Department of Veterans Affairs, June 3, 2015d. Available at: www.publichealth.va.gov/exposures/agentorange/conditions/index.asp. Accessed January 10, 2018.

U.S. Department of Veterans Affairs: Profile of Women Veterans: 2015. Washington, DC, U.S. Department of Veterans Affairs, December 2016a. Available at: www.va.gov/vetdata/docs/SpecialReports/Women_Veterans_Profile_12 22 2016.pdf. Accessed January 10, 2018.

U.S. Department of Veterans Affairs: VA Suicide Prevention Program Facts About Veteran Suicide. Washington, DC, U.S. Department of Veterans Affairs, July 2016b. Available at: www.va.gov/opa/publications/factsheets/Suicide_Prevention_FactSheet_New_VA_Stats_070616_1400.pdf. Accessed May 11, 2018.

U.S. Department of Veterans Affairs: Cold Injuries. Washington, DC, U.S. Department of Veterans Affairs, December 27, 2017. Available at: www.publichealth.va.gov/PUBLICHEALTH/exposures/cold-injuries/index.asp. Accessed January 10, 2018.

Wilson BA: Women Prisoners of War, 1996. Available at: http://userpages.aug.com/captbarb/prisoners.html. Accessed May 29, 2018.

Yaffe K, Vittinghoff E, Lindquist K, et al: Posttraumatic stress disorder and risk of dementia among US veterans. Arch Gen Psychiatry 67(6):608 613, 2010 20530010

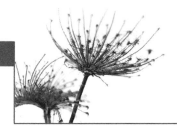

CHAPTER 1

1. True or False: Persons from ethnic minority groups are more likely than whites to interact with the health care system because minority elderly are more likely to have chronic illnesses.

    True.

2. True or False: For health care organizations, overall performance improvement is one of the benefits of providing culturally competent health care.

    True.

3. True or False: Regarding individual-level competence, ignoring implicit biases can improve hospital performance metrics.

    False.

4. True or False: In the context of health care provision, only direct communication needs to be addressed.

    True.

5. True or False: A recent American Heart Association study found that cardiovascular disease awareness among American women was significantly lower among Hispanics than whites.

    True.

6. Which of the following is *not* one of the main constructs in the Culturally Competent Model of Care?

   A. Cultural awareness.
   B. Cultural knowledge.
   C. Cultural stigma.
   D. Cultural encounters.
   E. Cultural desire.

   The correct response is option C.

CHAPTER 2

1. Name four essential practice-based learning and improvement techniques for cultural competence.

   Continued review of the medical literature, self-evaluation, educating others, and implementing quality improvement measures to provide more culturally competent care.

2. An elderly African American Vietnam era veteran has trauma-related symptoms of hypervigilance, anxiety, and nightmares that worsened in late life. A white psychiatry resident who is usually sympathetic with patients minimizes the effect of reported race baiting and threats by saying that the patient is just trying to get free benefits. In what ways does this vignette demonstrate unconscious biases that are affecting care?

   Acting "out of character" or being unable to empathize with the individual are key determinants indicating the presence of unconscious bias.

3. How might one learn about another culture without working directly with that group?

   Videos and literature profiling ethnic elderly, both positive models and pathological models, are often necessary to sensitize clinicians to a particular culture.

4. A work group tasked by the Association of Medical Colleges (AAMC) recommends how many curricular domains for cultural competency for medical students?

A. Three.
B. Five.
C. Eight.
D. Twelve.

The correct response is option A.

5. True or False: There is increased activation of the mentalizing areas of the brain during exposure of black faces to white subjects.

False.

CHAPTER 3

1. Which of the following are the three distinct stages of migration as identified by Bhugra and colleagues?

    A. Decision and preparation to migrate, physical relocation, and postmigration.
    B. Precontemplation, decision and preparation to migrate, and physical relocation.
    C. Decision and preparation to migrate, physical relocation, and acculturation.
    D. Decision and preparation to migrate, postmigration state, and adaptation.

The correct response is option A.

2. Which of the following stages of migration is associated with a relatively lower rate of mental illness and health problems?

    A. The migration process, involving actual physical relocation.
    B. The postmigration stage.
    C. The premigration stage.
    D. The precontemplation stage.

The correct response is option C.

3. Which of the following is a challenge that late-life immigrants encounter versus immigrants who came earlier in life?

A. Difficulty finding housing.

B. Difficulty obtaining public assistance.

C. Strenuous relationship with family members in the host country

D. Trouble communicating with loved ones in the country of birth.

The correct response is option B.

4. Among Medicare-eligible foreign-born elders, which of the following groups has the longest life expectancy due to high level of health on arrival, better health habits, and a strong social network?

A. Eastern Europeans.

B. Filipinos.

C. Blacks.

D. Cambodians.

E. Indians.

The correct response is option C.

5. What is the dual process of cultural and psychological change that takes place as a result of contact between two or more cultural groups and their individual members called?

A. Acculturation.

B. Immigration.

C. Migration.

D. Colonization.

The correct response is option A.

6. Match the following racial ethnic groups with the acculturation characteristics.

1. *African Caribbeans*   2. *Asians*   3. *Latinos*

A. Tridimensional acculturation paradigm.

B. Downward assimilation to inner-city African American culture.

C. Undocumented immigrant status, leading to reduced access to health care and other resources.

D. Settling in dense population enclaves, which may slow the process of acculturation.

E. Filial responsibility and parental authority core cultural beliefs that conflict with Western focus on individuality.

F. Nonhomogeneous group with varying socioeconomic, war, and political experiences affecting acculturation.

1: A, B; 2: E, F; 3: C, D.

7. Which mental disorder has a higher rate among immigrants, especially black immigrants?

A. Bipolar disorder.
B. Major depressive disorder.
C. Schizophrenia and psychosis.
D. Panic disorder.

The correct response is option C.

8. A 62-year-old Japanese American male presents to the psychiatrist with his daughter for evaluation. The daughter states that the patient moved to the United States 2 months ago. He has been irritable and complains of abdominal pain, knee pain, and headaches. He rarely smiles and constantly talks about his life back home. The patient does not speak English. Which measures should the psychiatrist take to ensure proper communication with the patient?

A. Allow the daughter to translate during the evaluation because she knows the patient best.
B. Bring in a nurse who reports that she speaks Japanese.
C. Use a professional translation service and use terms referring to the patient specifically.
D. Use Google Translate because it is the easiest way to obtain information.

The correct response is option C.

9. During the evaluation of older immigrants, which tools best help the clinician perform a more thorough assessment as a means to overcome cultural biases?

A. The Montreal Cognitive Assessment.
B. The Mini-Mental State Examination.

C. The Beck Depression Scale.

D. Scales measuring instrumental activities of daily living and everyday memory.

The correct response is option D.

10. Before prescribing a pharmacological agent to an elderly immigrant, it is most important that the clinician assess the use of indigenous healers, herbal remedies, the role of faith and religion, and which of the following?

A. Cytochrome P450 enzymes.

B. Patient's height.

C. Patient's level of education.

D. Patient's dentition.

The correct response is option A.

CHAPTER 4

1. According to the 2010 U.S. Census, what percentage of newly arrived immigrants have come from Asia?

A. 16%.

B. 26%.

C. 36%.

D. 46%.

The correct response is option C.

2. When elderly immigrant Asian Americans seek treatment for a medical illness, which of the following are they most likely to see first?

A. Community elder.

B. Primary care physician.

C. Hospital emergency department.

D. Traditional healer.

The correct response is option D.

3. Which of the following describes "semen loss?"

    A. *Dhat* syndrome.
    B. *Shenjing shuairuo.*
    C. *Hwa-byung.*
    D. *Khyâl cap.*

    The correct response is option A.

4. All of the following are traditional Asian healing methods used in the treatment of psychosis except

    A. Coining.
    B. Pinching.
    C. Cupping.
    D. Moxibustion.
    E. Sweat boxes.

    The correct response is option E.

5. Elderly immigrants from which of the following countries came primarily as political refugees?

    A. India.
    B. Vietnam.
    C. Singapore.
    D. South Korea.
    E. Japan.

    The correct response is option B.

6. Which of the following minority groups has the lowest incidence of dementia?

    A. Asian Americans.
    B. African Americans.
    C. Pacific Islanders.
    D. Alaska Natives.
    E. American Indians.

    The correct response is option A.

CHAPTER 5

1. Indigenous peoples after colonization had their culture and lands reduced as well as which of the following?

   A. Their languages were reduced from more than 300 distinct languages.
   B. They lost cultural practices and were banned from practicing their ceremonies for hundreds of years.
   C. Tribal groups were reduced from more than 15 million people to 3 million people.
   D. All of the above.

   The correct response is option D.

2. Intergenerational trauma in Indigenous peoples has been linked to various psychiatric issues, including which of the following?

   A. Lower rates of PTSD.
   B. Low IQ scores.
   C. High rates of attachment disorders.
   D. High rates of eating disorders.

   The correct response is option C.

3. True or False: Culture-bound syndromes (cultural concepts of distress in DSM-5) characterize the cultural influences on the expression and experience of mental disorders that can occur in a person.

   True.

4. Which cultural treatment modality has been effective with Indigenous elderly?

   A. Seeking out culturally appropriate healing ceremonies.
   B. Use of talking circles.
   C. Integrating Indigenous art and aesthetics into the Western medical clinical setting.
   D. A and C.
   E. All of the above.

   The correct response is option E.

CHAPTER 6

1. West African health traditions reflect a holistic ideology in which good health is the result of a harmonious relationship with nature and man and disease is classified under all of the following headings except

    A. Natural.
    B. Occult.
    C. Spiritual.
    D. Traditional.

    The correct response is option D.

2. True or False: The U.S. Public Health Service's Tuskegee Study of Untreated Syphilis enrolled 600 African Americans, promising free health care and death benefits, but resulted in many subjects progressing through the full course of untreated syphilis, ultimately ending in their death.

    True.

3. True or False: Older African Americans are more likely than older whites to perceive cognitive impairment as a normal part of aging.

    True.

4. Compared with white caregivers of older adults with neurocognitive impairment, African American caregivers are more likely to demonstrate which of the following?

    A. Depression.
    B. Anxiety.
    C. Hostility.
    D. Resourcefulness.

    The correct response is option D.

CHAPTER 7

1. True or False: Latino elders are a homogenous group, and the one and only common thread is that they speak Spanish.

   False.

2. Latino culture has three normative values that must be recognized in any clinical setting. List these values.

   Simpatía **(kindness),** *personalismo* **(friendliness),** *respeto* **(respect).**

3. True or False: Suicide rates among all Latino elderly immigrants are generally low.

   False.

4. Strategies for creating a culturally sensitive environment for Latino patients include which of the following?

   A. Allowing extra time for patients with limited English proficiency.
   B. Posting bilingual or Spanish language signage.
   C. Providing culturally sensitive training for staff.
   D. All of the above.

   The correct response is option D.

CHAPTER 8

1. The range believed to best reflect the number of older LGBT individuals in the United States is

   A. 100,000–500,000
   B. 1–3 million
   C. 10–20 million
   D. 25–50 million
   E. More than 50 million

   The correct response is option B.

2. Which statement is true regarding sex, gender identity, and gender expression?

    A. Gender expression is always the same as one's sex.
    B. Gender identity is always the same as one's sex.
    C. Research has demonstrated that there is no reason to discard a binary understanding of gender identity.
    D. Sex is the term used to identify a newborn as either male or female.
    E. These are synonymous terms used at birth to identify a newborn as either male or female.

The correct response is option D.

3. Which of the following statements best describes intersectionality?

    A. By ignoring a person's membership in an older age cohort, intersectionality improves one's understanding of a person's identity.
    B. Intersectionality is a concept that discourages the development of diversity-informed case conceptualizations.
    C. Intersectionality is the term recently developed to describe the ability of members of gender or sexual minorities to interact with individuals who do not belong to a gender or sexual minority.
    D. Intersectionality is the term used to describe the odds that a member of a gender or sexual minority will meet another member of the same minority.
    E. Intersectionality requires that an individual be viewed as more than the sum of his or her parts or any one personal identity marker such as age, race, or sexual orientation.

The correct response is option E.

4. Which of the following statements is true regarding the experiences and challenges of older members of the LGBT community?

    A. Data from the New York City Department of Health and Mental Hygiene found that lesbian and bisexual women were only about 10% more likely than heterosexual women to live alone.

B. Data from the New York City Department of Health and Mental Hygiene showed that gay and bisexual men older than 50 were much less likely than heterosexual men to be living alone.

C. When an older LGBT adult has been living out of the closet and then moves into residential care, going back into the closet is rarely a decision that seems reasonable.

D. The older the LGBT individual, the more likely that the individual has been impacted by minority stress.

E. The older the LGBT individual, the less likely that the individual has been impacted by minority stress.

The correct response is option D.

CHAPTER 9

1. True or False: Demographic features of rural America may be characterized as predominantly white and agricultural consistently over the past decade.

   False

2. National trends regarding substance abuse suggest which of the following is true in rural populations?

   A. Substance use rates are increasing in older adults.

   B. Older adults in rural areas display lower rates of substance use than urban adults.

   C. Rural areas are demonstrating stable rates of substance use among both young and older adults.

   The correct response is option A.

3. Which of the following describes a problem for rural adults in seeking mental health care?

   A. Reduced availability of specialty care, particularly for dementia.

   B. High rates of stigma toward psychiatric services.

   C. Increased isolation due to geographic barriers.

   D. All of the above.

   The correct response is option D.

4. Which of the following providers is most likely to perform dementia evaluations in rural settings?

    A. Geriatric psychiatrist.
    B. Social worker.
    C. Primary care provider.
    D. Psychologist.
    E. Neurologist.

    The correct response is option C.

5. Which of the following is more likely to be true of rural residents when compared with their urban counterparts?

    A. They have higher educational attainment.
    B. They are ethnically diverse.
    C. They have full-time, high-paying jobs.
    D. They receive Social Security benefits.

    The correct response is option D.

CHAPTER 10

1. True or False: Behavior plays a larger role than genetics in reaching the age of 80.

    True.

2. True or False: Behavior plays a larger role than genetics in reaching an age beyond 90.

    False.

3. True or False: Among centenarians, the personality configuration of low neuroticism, high competence, and high extraversion traits is overrepresented relative to chance.

    True.

CHAPTER 11

1. Most present-day veterans served during which of the following eras?

   A. World War II.
   B. Korean War.
   C. Vietnam.
   D. First Gulf War.
   E. Operation Enduring Freedom/Operation Iraqi Freedom.

   The correct response is option C.

2. Which of the following combat occupational exposures has been associated with an increased risk of developing dementia in a 9-year follow-up period?

   A. Mustard gas.
   B. Agent Orange.
   C. Exposure to cold.
   D. Traumatic brain injury.
   E. Extreme physical activity.

   The correct response is option D.

3. True or False: In later life, all veterans who stop consuming alcohol demonstrate improved quality of life and fewer psychological symptoms.

   False.

4. True or False: As combat veterans age and develop dementia, symptoms of PTSD can recur.

   True.

5. Which of the following medications has been found to decrease nightmares associated with PTSD?

   A. Propranolol.
   B. Cimetidine.
   C. Amantadine.

D. Prazocin.

E. Quetiapine.

The correct response is option D.

6. All of the following items are risk factors for suicide among active duty service members except

A. Relationship difficulties.

B. Access to firearms.

C. Pain.

D. Occupational problems.

E. Fear of death.

The correct response is option E.

Index

*Page numbers printed in **boldface** type refer to tables or figures*